About th

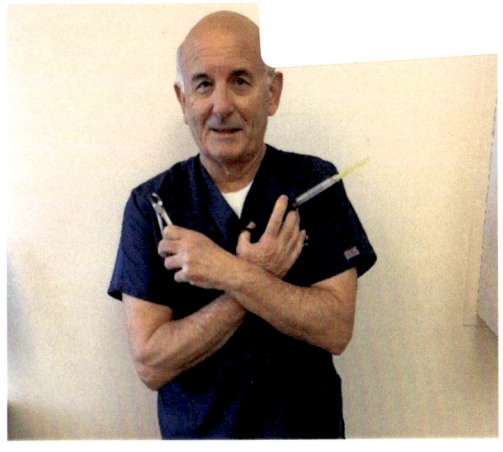

In my early teens, I knew I wanted to become a dentist. Working in the NHS and the private sector, I enjoyed all aspects of a unique profession. My wife, Sue, has been tremendously supportive in this project, together with my three children. I found that fishing on my local river for trout and salmon helped me through difficult times, a hobby that continues to this day. Growing vegetables and teaching karate, as a fifth dan black belt instructor, have also provided valuable relaxation. As I approach retirement, I can look back at some wonderful memories that are worth sharing, recalling the people I have met along my chosen path. All that has enriched my life.

OPEN WIDE!
FIFTY GLORIOUS YEARS AS A DENTIST

Dr Bernard Lester BDS (U.Manc) MJDF RCS

OPEN WIDE!
FIFTY GLORIOUS YEARS AS A
DENTIST

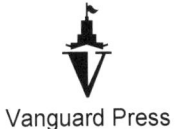

Vanguard Press

A CIP catalogue record for this title is
available from the British Library.

ISBN 978-1-80016-023-1

*Vanguard Press is an imprint of
Pegasus Elliot MacKenzie Publishers Ltd.*
www.pegasuspublishers.com

First Published in 2021

**Vanguard Press
Sheraton House Castle Park
Cambridge England**

Printed & Bound in Great Britain

Dedication

To my wonderful wife, Sue, and children,
Sarah, Andrew and Rebecca, without whom
life would be meaningless.
To my parents, Ena and Joe, for giving me the
opportunity and freedom to choose my
career.
To my in-laws, Sophia and Maurice, for their
constant support.
Also, to my brothers, Rik and Phil, for being
there.

Acknowledgements

My wife, Sue, constant companion and source of inspiration. My very dear colleague, Gary Simon, for all the ups and downs we have shared together and a friendship that has lasted all my life. All the students in the year of '69 who made my university days so special. My wonderful staff who have put up with me throughout my professional life. The long list of patients who have made this memoir worth writing.

Roger Williams whose advice and support was invaluable, and all my other dear colleagues at the St. John Street Medical Association, who were a constant source of experience and wisdom.

Andrew Morrell, President Cobra Martial Arts, for trying to keep me in shape.

Contents

Chapter One
In the Beginning

Oh no, not the dentist. A visit to that scary person who had all those instruments of torture at his fingertips in a room that smelled disgusting. Can you remember the fear as a child? I can! My mother didn't tell me in advance where we were going until that fateful day of my very first visit. From my classmates I had heard all the stories of drills and pain—I felt physically sick.

I remember sitting on a hard bench, waiting, then my name was called. The antiseptic smell, the blinding light above, and that chair that had all sorts of instruments attached to it, each I thought capable of inflicting pain. There was the tinkle of the instruments on the cold looking table while the boiler bubbled away like a witch's cauldron. Then I had to sit down in the chair that seemed to have a life of its own: it moved, it lifted me up, it was hard and impersonal. Keep statue-still and open wide. No anaesthetic, a slow drill.

"Just a little more," he lied. Finally, the filling was completed—relief for six whole months.

"Would you like a sweet?" the nurse said on the way out.

So, who would want to be a dentist? Well, me actually. Despite my first experience, the trauma turned into ambition. I was going to be the dentist who would change perceptions of the Dracula figure. You might find reasons to avoid me, but I knew I would be able to inspire confidence and trust. I was going to shatter the stereotype.

As you'll see later, my philosophy has been in line with Rudyard Kipling's famous lines: *If you can meet with triumph and disaster and treat those two imposters just the same*. Believe me, I have faced both in my career. After fifty years in dentistry, I am certainly now triumphant, sitting on a glorious Indian Ocean beach, gathering my memories for this book, far away from the surgery, contemplating retirement.

I want to tell you what it is like to be a dentist: the laughter, the wonderful interaction with people who trust you implicitly, the successes and failures, and of course, the stress. My first tutor once joked that if patients just handed in their teeth for repair and said, "I will collect them tomorrow, Doc", it would be an easy profession. In a way that is precisely what did happen in the dark ages, but thankfully, we've moved on.

From the age of thirteen I knew that I wanted to become a dentist. But why? My father was a teacher, my mother a machinist, so no following in footsteps there. But maybe this memory of a conversation with a school friend, Gary, might provide an answer.

It went something like this:

Me: What are we going to do when we finish school?

Friend: We're only thirteen. Anyway, I want to be a pop star.

Me: Tempting, but you can't sing or play an instrument.

Friend: Fair point. What about a gynaecologist?

Me: Only an amateur!

Friend: Is that all you think about?

Me: Well, maybe Bridget Bardot needs a new manager.

Friend: Is that all you think about?

Me: Not all, I support Manchester City.

Friend: Yes, well they need all the support they can get.

Me: Fair point.

Friend: What about a footballer?

Me: But you play for the scraps! (A colloquialism for the people who don't make any team.)

Friend: Fair point.

Me: There must be something we can get our teeth into… That's it! Let's fill teeth!

Friend: Okay, they only need three A level passes, any grade.

Me: Fair point.

I remember vividly the day we caught the bus to school heading for the office to collect our A-level results, hearts thumping, minds racing. What do we do if we fail? For us it was dentistry or nothing, with the only other option to open a bar on a distant beach; however, it was pointed out to us that we were not old enough to buy alcohol let alone sell it. No fears, we both passed with flying colours and we were now dental students.

So that's how it all started.

What follows is an honest account of the trials and tribulations and hilarious times of a boy, a student and a dental surgeon in a profession that I love.

Chapter Two
First Day

Here we were at the magnificent Manchester Medical School, where the future doctors and dentists embarked on their respective courses. My friend and I were late, of course, but made our way to the small lecture theatre where we were to begin to discover the mysteries of anatomy and physiology. I opened the door and crept in quietly. Unfortunately, I missed a stair, tripped and became the centre of attention. Our senior anatomy tutor, Dr Tanner, a diminutive man but with an aura of a serene dictator, could make you sit up and listen with just a stare. "Welcome!" he said. "Now sit down and make sure that is your only accident in this building." Laughter all round! Suitably embarrassed and chastened I sat and listened to the introduction.

"Now," Dr Tanner announced, "we have divided you into six groups of six and you will begin your anatomy practical. Please go through into the dissection room."

We trooped in, all smiles and bravado, into a room with six tables, each covered by a sheet with what appeared to be a cadaver underneath. Gerry, who eventually turned into our resident comedian, gasped then emitted a loud, "Oh shit, no!"

We grouped around our dissection bodies with our tutors who lifted the sheets in an orchestrated manner, as if revealing a gourmet dish, to expose our formalin pickled cadavers. Now we were eighteen to nineteen years old, naive and shocked. After thirty seconds the place looked like A and E on a bad night, with most of the students fainting or retching. Then suddenly there was a scream from Amy at the back table. "What's that?" she yelled in horror, staring at a procedure being conducted by one of the senior tutors.

"I'm examining the blood vessels of the penis," he replied. "It's the only time I have to get my anatomy dissection completed."

Amy ran out in tears and it took some persuading to encourage her to return to the lab sometime later.

Once we had finally adapted to the task of dissection, after each anatomy session a group of us with strong stomachs would troop off to the local greasy spoon opposite the medical school for a curry. The general idea was that the smell of the curry disguised the aroma of formalin. Depending on the curry on the day, this generally worked.

These wonderful people who donated their bodies for medical research were always treated with the utmost respect, but as students, to be confronted with a human body was the most surreal event of our days at the hospital. There was, however, one exception. One medical student who looked like he was always on the verge of a nervous breakdown, a real loner, suddenly in the common room produced a dissected finger and shouted, "I've won! I've won!". We never saw him again and always wondered what had happened to him. Some years later, I saw him on TV, having developed a career in politics.

Our intrepid group of thirty-three gradually gelled into what was generally considered to be the best set of characters the school had seen. Well, we thought so anyway. As we faced the challenges of our first year, we became a mutually supportive community and developed a camaraderie that lasted for many years after we qualified. Most of us overcame the first hurdle, the anatomy and physiology exams; those who didn't retook them the following year.

Suddenly it began, what we had been eagerly awaiting. Real dentistry. We moved into the dental school clad in our crisp white coats. How proud we were strutting around with our conservation kits, the beautiful wooden boxes each containing a set of drawers which housed all of the instruments we would use to practise on our innocent patients. The contents looked as if they came from the Spanish Inquisition but hey, we were becoming dentists. After fifty years I still have my box. I use it now to store my trout and salmon fishing flies.

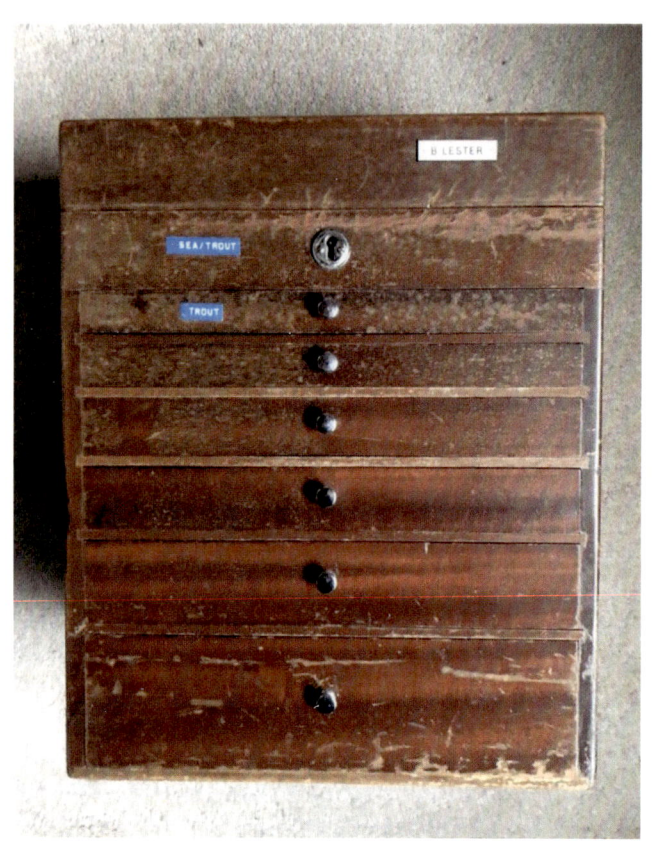

Chapter 3
Real Dental Students

The next three years were the happiest of my days in education. I had met my wife-to-be Sue on my first day in freshers' week though she wasn't a dental student. As an arts student she had only a minimal number of lectures and seminars per week, whereas we were working flat out five days a week and with relatively short holidays. Student life was very different for us but belonging to a small group of colleagues had fantastic advantages, both socially and professionally. Friendships were made and cemented in the common room and in the surgeries. We did manage to have a lot of fun.

My friend, Don, and I became table football champions and remained unbeaten. Pep, eat your heart out. As we were both Manchester City supporters it was our golden age, Lee, Bell and Summerbee. We were unbeaten at canasta, admittedly by means of cheating. We referred to City players' numbers as a code to collecting cards, an offence only admitted at our fortieth reunion. All this as well as living through the sixties.

Life was purposeful and uncluttered, apart from the stress of examinations.

Sometimes things happen in life that cannot be scripted. Our benign anatomy dictator and tutor, Doctor Tanner, suddenly decided that he had had enough of the politics in his department, and thought it might be a good idea if he joined our year and become a dentist. The rumour spread like gonorrhoea in a brothel. Lo and behold it was true, and just after we had all passed our anatomy exams, he joined us as a student.

"Wait just a minute," I dared to challenge him. "You haven't passed your anatomy examination yet."

He dissolved in laughter and retorted, "You may test me at your leisure." To his credit he became and was accepted as one of the students and was elected as honorary president of our year. At our twenty-fifth reunion, whilst making a speech, my opening line was that even after twenty-five years, he still scared the shit out of me.

We started on dental anatomy, which had an eighty per cent failure rate, then progressed to conservation (fillings), prosthetics (dentures), pathology and bacteriology (path and bugs), and the dreaded oral surgery.

My first filling done in amalgam was completed on what we called a phantom head. This was a set of plastic teeth set in just that, a wooden phantom head. I began by drilling a cavity with a slow handpiece, no fancy high speed ones that we use today. Then there was the lining and finally the amalgam filling was pressed in place. Once this skill had been mastered, progression was to filling a previously extracted tooth set in plaster. I still have my first filling done this way, which must have fallen into my white coat pocket.

Now it's okay doing all these fiddly fillings on a plastic model, but then it was real patients. We were set free on the public. Each stage was carefully checked before being signed off, and we were given points depending on the size of the filling. Strangely this system resembled what it was like after qualification, except we were paid in points instead of pounds. We were shown how to give injections, wow now I'm a real dentist (triumph!).

It was then the turn of the patients in oral surgery (OS) to witness my sensational skills. Surely there had never been a better dentist than me? My first extraction bought me down to earth with a clatter. The OS department, in my opinion, was run by some of the most liked and disliked people in the hospital because they were so competitive, jousting for the top jobs constantly. Miss Gee, an instructor in Oral Surgery, looked at me, smiled and said, "Lester, go into cubicle one and complete the case." At the same time, she managed to glare at me as if Frankenstein himself was in the cubicle. (As it happens there really was a very good dentist called Frankenstein.) I walked confidently into the room to be confronted by a six-foot three-inch giant of a man built like Desperate Dan. Now I am five foot six, so I felt a little easier when he sat down in the chair.

"Take this lower tooth out, Doc, as quick as you can. I've got to get back to work on the building site across the road." This was said with alcohol fuelled bravado.

"Okay," I replied, glancing at the medical history. No problems there. Bugger, I thought. This will need a lower nerve block (ID). Not the easiest of injections, as you have to position the needle so that as it passes through the tissue at the back of the mouth where it touches the bone of the mandible, the lower jaw. Hard enough for an experienced practitioner; for me almost impossible. The first attempt missed and I felt that it probably anaesthetised an area somewhere below the chin, possibly in the neck. I reloaded and hit the spot.

Now we had to wait five minutes, which was how I learnt about the patient's colourful past: his three marriages, the shooting in Nigeria, where he insisted in showing me the scar in his left buttock.

Time for the extraction. I chose the correct forceps and applied 'buccal pressure,' (towards the cheek). We were always told to adopt this principle when extracting a lower molar. I could not move it even with one foot off the ground. So, I called in Miss Gee who was still smirking, and explained that I could not budge the tooth.

"Try moving it lingually, boy," (towards the tongue) she instructed.

"But I was told to move it buccally," I protested.

"Who told you that?"

"Well, actually you did," I stammered. I saw my whole past life flash in front of me. Gee was apoplectic and stormed out.

"Do as you want, Doc," interrupted the patient, unfazed by the trauma. I tried again and did as Gee said, and lo and behold out popped the tooth and no fracture.

"Fuck me," he said. "I think the roots went straight down to my balls."

'Close,' I thought.

I dismissed the patient who, in a very loud voice, announced that I was, "The best dentist in Manchester." I think this must have been the four pints of beer talking. However, I was still shaking and accepted the plaudits. As I walked past the other students who had stopped to listen to the drama, Gerry, so that Miss Gee and the other students could hear, said calmly, "Well done, Bernie. I think you can risk a fart now." (Triumph!).

My first attempted filling on a real person, however, did not go so well. I went to the waiting room to collect my patient and introduce myself. I was confronted by a woman in her early twenties looking very apprehensive. I took her to my dental unit, glanced at the notes and told her I was going to give her a local anaesthetic, which made her paler still. The tutor, who had spotted her distress came over to reassure her.

The patient looked up at him: "I would rather have a baby than a filling."

The tutor, in his most professional voice replied, "Well, miss, make up your mind before he adjusts the chair. He has tools for both jobs, you know." The poor lady put her hand to her mouth to stifle a scream, jumped out of the chair, ran down the corridor and out of the building. I wrote on the record card 'patient declined treatment'. (Disaster).

Next patient, please!

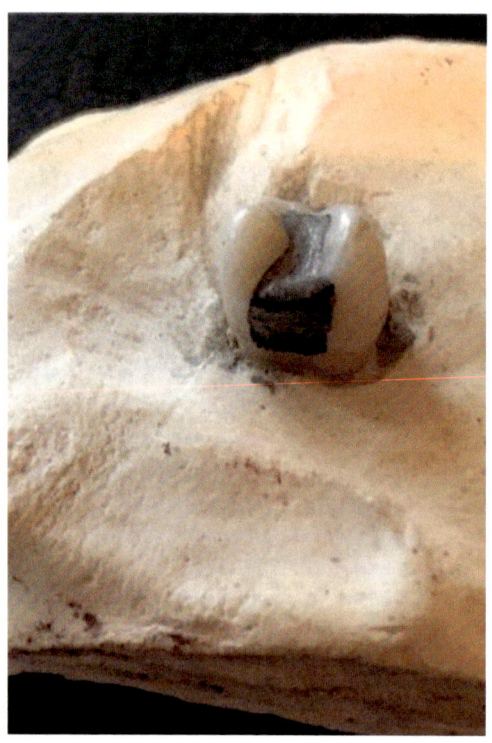

First filling on a tooth set in plaster

Chapter Four
Four Fun Years

Our days in the dental school were filled with the wonder of learning new procedures. We made crowns in real gold, extracted teeth and I completed my first fixed bridge—two crowns supporting an extra tooth to fill a gap. The patient, who was getting married shortly after the treatment, looked in the mirror, turned around and kissed me passionately. Now this was in front of several students and tutors so I felt safe. Shortly after I received a wedding invitation and the most wonderful thank you card, which I have kept to this day. (Triumph.)

One of the most challenging areas of dentistry is prosthetics, making false teeth. As students we were responsible for constructing each stage ourselves. Once qualified and in practice, a technician would do this for us. After initial impressions, we would make a wax bite block to make sure the occlusion (meeting) of the teeth was correct, then carefully add the teeth to a wax template. At this stage we would try the teeth into the patient's mouth so they could look in a mirror and, if satisfactory, we would finish them off in acrylic resin.

My first full denture case was a rough looking man with a heart of gold, who insisted in bringing chocolates and biscuits at every visit. At the try in stage, he looked in the mirror and in a loud voice announced, "Bloody perfect, Doc!" Whilst I was finding the tutor to sign off the stage, the patient left with the accolade, "You are the best thing since sliced bread and should be by appointment to the queen". (Triumph!). Unfortunately, we could not find him before he disappeared, to explain that the teeth were only set, in wax. After an hour we received a phone call to say that all the teeth had fallen out, he was not going to come back to see that charlatan again, and that I should be struck off. (Disaster.)

Our examination in prosthetics (dentures) was particularly difficult because we had to design a chrome-cobalt metal plate in wax, showing the extension and where the clasps were to be placed. This was a task that we always left to our tutors and technicians. Strangely, the day before we were due to take the exam, one of the denture technicians left a complete mock-up of what we had to complete in the common room. We all eagerly took mental notes and then destroyed the evidence. We all passed with flying colours and thereafter he always received a bottle of wine at Christmas. The senior tutor said it was remarkable that we had all used the same design, and he thought that this was a tribute to the department teaching. (Typical, taking the credit.)

As a 'now for something completely different', it was decided that we all needed a lecture on contraception. What did they think we students were up to? Well, it was the swinging sixties. There we were, grouped in the lecture theatre, where the local family planning nurse did her best to keep a straight face. "I always thought that dentists couldn't fill any cavities below the neck," was her opening line, whilst at the same time she tried to put a condom on a banana. We then had to practise on various sized bananas. (Disaster!)

More seriously, every Wednesday, we were closeted in a darkened room to discuss X-rays and diagnoses, which was more like the back row of the local cinema. On one occasion, Gerry fell asleep and was left there until the caretaker woke him up.

One highlight towards the end of my final year was when I actually won the MacLean's Children's Prize for Dentistry, mainly for my ability to treat very difficult children and get them not only to sit on the chair, but to have treatment. This accomplishment always amazed the tutors, who had been unable to treat these patients themselves; they concluded that I was going to be a gifted paediatric (children's) dentist. In fact, my success was due to the fact that I had taken advice from a senior qualified colleague, who suggested that if the scally would not agree to treatment—and remember we saw some of the most unruly, and badly behaved children— I should gently whisper in the child's ear,' If you don't get on the chair and go along with treatment, I'll nail your... ears to the headrest!' Strangely worked like a charm. A technique dropped after qualification.

Amidst all of the traumas with patients, relationships were always going to cause problems for the students. Remember, we were segregated from the main university, so it became very insular. However, some relationships stayed the course and some couples married as students or after qualification. So that contraception lecture wasn't completely wasted.

Chapter Five
Finals, Oh No!

On my first day at university, I met my favourite lady, Sue. We had planned to get married three months after finals. No pressure, then! I needed to become a responsible, professional husband.

Our final exams were spread over two weeks in November 1969 and covered every subject. This was a frantic, incredibly stressful time for us all, but as a group we were determined to confront the examiners. There were written papers, practicals on teeth and, of course, the dreaded vivas and spotters. For these last, various specimens were placed in cubicles and we were to go from one to another then explain to the examiner what they were. Terrifying!

"No, Mr Collier, it is not a piece of curried chicken, it's a portion of the brain." This loud pronouncement was just what was needed to relieve the tension.

During one of the spotters, I `accidentally` dropped a chocolate Smartie on a section of heart. Gerry, who was behind me, was asked by the examiner for his comments on the specimen. After looking it over carefully, in a most impressive and professional voice, he pronounced, "Obviously it`s a bad case of a cute smart attack." The examiner turned away, either in exasperation or more likely to stop himself laughing.

My last exam was at eight-thirty on a Friday morning. It was potentially the most difficult as it involved peering through microscopes and identifying what tissue was on the slide. Now my dear father was president of the Manchester Microscopic Society, so I had access to microscopes at home whenever I needed. In this exam I excelled.

The examiner said to me, "As a dentist, what is your view of..." Had I misheard? Did he actually address me as 'dentist'? I cannot remember what he asked me but it was then that I realised that I might have finally realised my dream. (Triumph!)

After my turn, DP, who always followed me in exams, whispered that I always gave him confidence. If he only knew what stomach churning my anxieties had put me through.

After the final examinations, as we waited for the results to be published that afternoon, a group of us went to the Gaumont cinema, close to the dental hospital, in the hope of distraction. Some watched *The Dirty Dozen*; some slept through it; others looked at the screen and cried as if it was some form of anaesthetic, which indeed it was. To this day, the film will always have a special place in my psyche, and whenever it has been shown again it brings back those memories. At four p.m. the news spread along the rows in hushed tones: 'The results will be out now.'

So, this was it. Four and a half years at university and I had wanted to become a dentist since I was thirteen. I stared at the noticeboard and there it was: *The following have satisfied the examiners.* Well, I know one lady student who might have, and I don't mean in the exams, but that's another tale and not important now.

I scanned the board and there it was. My name in black type on white paper. Halleluiah, I really had passed. (Triumph!)

Such was the impact of final examinations on me, I still have surreal nightmares about them, a recurring theme of being in a church going to confession. For a Jewish boy this is a little odd. The dream follows the same scenario where the father confessor tells me I'm going to fail because of all my sins. The only way to deal with it is to recite three Hail Marys and the whole Megillah, a Jewish prayer.

·

Chapter Six
My God! A Wife and a Mortgage

Man plans, God laughs! I thought Sue and I could spend six months travelling after the wedding, and before that I planned that I would have three months sitting around the common room with my friends, drinking, smoking and generally making nuisances of ourselves. But no. On a routine visit to my own dentist in Crumpsall, Brian reminded me that I had promised to join him as an associate dentist as soon as I had qualified. Whoops! I forgot. Possibly! Surely not?

Patients who thought that I knew it all, with nobody leaning over my shoulder to check my work. Student to dentist. Any chance of an interlude? But marriage and mortgage loomed.

And so it began. I started work and got my first mortgage for a house that actually we still live in today. But there was so much still to learn about and pay for. Dental indemnity protection, General Dental Council, British Dental Association fees, it was already adding up. Brian was kind enough to advance me a small payment as I was stony broke now that my grant had stopped.

I was still living in my parents' home as I was not yet married, but on my first day at work, a dismal dark rainy day in January, I was late. It is hard to explain the effect of this sudden change in my life, from a relatively carefree student to a professional, weighed down with debt, expenses and real responsibility. This was a time of crisis in my life and it took me six months before I came to terms with this sudden transition. It was a time that I really experienced some modicum of depression; the sudden wrenching from student to dentist with commitments, affected me considerably. It wasn't just me because this was a familiar trait amongst my contemporaries.

And so, on my first day I arrived late and was informed by Mrs Warner, the receptionist, that I had twelve patients to see. I did not realise that they had all arrived at the same time, however.

My first patient, a simple extraction, or so I thought. The tooth fractured; not negligence—it can happen. It is a requirement to inform the patient and plan future treatment. I struggled through my first morning in a state of shock as I had never before seen so many patients in one session. Welcome to the NHS.

My first patient in the afternoon was an extraction of an upper wisdom tooth. I took an X-ray and all seemed straightforward. On the record card it said 'No LA' (no local anaesthetic requested). Really? I duly chose the correct forceps and took the tooth out. (Triumph!) Ruth, my nurse, who viewed associates as something less than human excrement, gasped and her jaw dropped. The patient, who had been wonderful so far, decided, "I think I will have an anaesthetic next time." 'No LA' on the records meant no anaesthetic requested for fillings, not extractions. (Disaster!) Live and learn, Bernard.

The next three months were the most difficult of my career. It's one thing knowing the theory behind the various treatments, but now I was expected to put them into practice. However, I slowly became acquainted with the patients; some actually knew me as I used to live quite close to the surgery, and guess what, most actually liked my style. Talking to the patients made me understand their fears and expectations of treatment and enabled me to put them at ease. So, I'm not a humane killer. (Triumph.)

Then one day a letter arrived marked personal. This is it, I thought, my first legal letter claiming that I had been negligent, or assaulted a patient and caused them harm. The awful sinking feeling returned to fuel my anxieties. Now that's my under-confident self, talking. No, it was from the mother of a patient, saying, 'Dear Mr Lester—' no doctor then, "My daughter came in for treatment yesterday and was very impressed with your treatment and found you very amiable. I would like to know if you would consider a relationship with her leading to marriage." How was I supposed to reply? I spoke to my boss who calmly reassured me that similar things had happened to him. "Just write back saying thank you, but you are already engaged." This seemed to settle the situation as I never saw her again. I never told my soon to be wife, but I will feel awkward if she reads this.

My last patient before my marriage was an odd one. Brian asked me to see a patient of his as he had an emergency to see, which made me a little suspicious. Fair enough, I thought, and called Ms M into the surgery. The patient was an attractive woman in her mid-twenties, wearing a worryingly short skirt.

"Hello," I said, "what is the problem?"

"Well," she replied, and promptly lifted her skirt. "Can you look at my navel it's a little sore?"

The nurse, 'she who must be obeyed', stifled a laugh. Completely thrown for a moment, I did manage to come up with, "I'm sorry, it's a little low for my field."

No wonder the boss had passed her over to me. The patient, it seemed, had a habit of exposing herself in various situations and was well known in the area. We settled for an examination of her mouth instead.

Chapter Seven
General Anaesthetics (GA)

At this time, we were allowed to use a combination of nitrous oxide (laughing gas), oxygen plus a little halothane to anaesthetise patients for extractions. No appointments were needed; people just came in for the first few hours four mornings a week. We had another dentist giving the anaesthetic while I did the extractions. Nowadays no general anaesthetics are allowed to be given in a dental surgery. These times were not a highlight of my career. Most of the patients were children and this was a heart-rending experience for me. Such was the general state of children's teeth at that time it was the only answer for children who were suffering. I can remember now those little hands I used to hold during the procedure and the genuine fear in their eyes. Often, I found this too upsetting and had to excuse myself from the surgery.

Fortunately, general anaesthetics were phased out soon after I started, and I endeavoured to educate the parents more with diet and oral hygiene, together with regular attendance. As you will see, this worked well and improved the general dental health of the children I saw.

Sometimes patients lost bladder control with a GA and urinated during the procedure. As well as being embarrassing for the patient, this was not an easy job for the nursing staff, because the dental chairs at that time had cavity areas under them. The urine can collect inside and on one fateful Monday morning, I can remember tipping the chair back, and yes, Friday's urine spilt out over my legs and the nurse's feet. Not a very fragrant start to the week.

After nine months my boss called me into his surgery with news: "Bernard, I'm leaving the surgery, I want to sell up. Are you interested?"

Let's look at this situation. In the space of one year, I qualified, married and started working in the NHS. From being a carefree student, life and the real world suddenly hit me and I had to make this major decision, whether to buy out the surgery I had been going to as a boy, or let the chance pass. I talked to my family, friends and contemporaries and they all agreed this was an opportunity too good to pass up. Fate, destiny or karma, I had to accept.

Chapter Eight
Life in the NHS: My First Practice

It is called the business of dentistry for a reason. The bank would only lend me half of the amount needed, and I had to pay Brian the remainder over the next two years. However, it all went through and I was the proud owner of my own surgery after only nine months in practice. Phew! Now I had to put claim forms into the NHS in order to get paid, I had wages to pay, materials to purchase, rates and laboratory fees. All took a large chunk from my income. The property was an old house with rooms that I had never been into, but hey, they were my rooms, in my surgery, the surgery that I originally went to as a child.

Slowly I brought in my own staff. Many stayed with me for all the time that I remained in the NHS, and as I took over, 'she who must be obeyed' left. (Triumph) My trusted technician, Bret, did everything he could to help me build the practice and we shared many years of a good partnership. Now I was able to do the sort of dentistry that really helped the community. Yes, I did the usual routine aspects of dentistry, but what worked was to have a good rapport with the patients. I had the most wonderful staff now and they worked hard to make the surgery a focus for oral health education. We gave prizes to the children, started a monthly magazine, and asked the patients for suggestions. Most were very constructive. (The odd one, anonymous, used to make lewd comments about the staff.) All my plans were in place, the surgery was full, I was enjoying my dentistry, but then an increase in charges paid by the patients was introduced dictated by the government. Instead of one pound fifty standing charge, it was increased to ten pounds. (Disaster!)

This, I thought, was catastrophic, the end of my short career, bank mortgage, bank loan, bank overdraft, bankrupt.

On the Wednesday before the new charges came into effect, known in my surgery as 'Black Wednesday', we saw eighty-one patients. I do not remember going home, but when I saw my trusted nurse Susan, she had her head in her hands and begged me, "Please, no more patients," so at ten p.m. we finished and locked up.

As the new charges filtered through there was a drop off in patient numbers but not, as I thought, significant. Just as we were settling back into a routine, the miners' strike happened. (Disaster). In the middle of surgery, the power would suddenly go off. No lights, so what did we do? We improvised. Strapped torches to the unit and set up as many battery powered lights as we could get hold of to give us a modicum of normality.

The surgery resembled a fairy grotto. We struggled through in the end with very little disruption. (Success.)

Now I was doing crowns and bridges and all the constructive parts of dentistry that I had hoped to do. Make no mistake, though, it was hard work. There were serious pressures, financial and personal. I was beginning to show signs of stress and distress, noticed by the staff as well as my dear wife, Sue. She decided we needed a holiday so we trooped off to Cornwall for a week to recharge the batteries. This was in the nick of time because I think just then I was heading for serious mental problems, mainly caused by the sudden changes in my life—work, a surgery, a mortgage—all of which had turned my life upside down. Welcome to the real world.

When I returned, I felt much better, but I was stony broke. As if there had been some divine intervention a patient paid her bill for my first private treatment. What joy, we could eat. This blip in my customary stable mental condition was a real lesson. These sudden life changes, coupled with financial and business stresses, combined to really knock me off track for a while. It was recognition of the issues and the support of my family and friends that made me come to terms with my problems; knowing what the cause is will always help with the cure.

Although these holidays proved therapeutic, I realised that whenever I managed to take two weeks' holiday, the first week was literally winding down and destressing. Three days before returning to work I was already worrying about what I would find when I was back at the surgery. This was mostly due to my personality traits, in that I cared about my profession and the patients A few weeks later I was back on track and the surgery was back in the old routine.

Now, it is good practice that when we see a patient for the first time, or a recall, we do a soft tissue check; now I would call it a mouth cancer check. We check for swollen glands in the head and neck and look for any sinister lesions. On a beautiful spring morning in 1973, I saw a middle-aged patient, Mrs W, for the first time. She was a heavy smoker and had a high alcohol consumption; this would always put you on red alert. I examined the tongue and sure enough there was an indurated (hardened) lesion about a centimetre in diameter on the left lateral side. I explained to her that I was unsure of the cause and promptly referred her to the local hospital. Two months later I received a letter from the hospital confirming my diagnosis of a squamous cell carcinoma of the tongue, cancer, and they had operated to remove it. Shortly after I received another letter from the patient thanking me for 'saving her life'. (Triumph.) But sadly, we found out a year later she had died from spread of the cancer. (Disaster.) We were all very subdued when we heard the news. This was the first, but not the last time that I had to refer people to hospital for investigation, but not always with such a tragic outcome. Often, if caught in time, the treatment will be successful.

Now for something completely different.

Mr J came to see me as a new patient, complaining of sensitive teeth. I commenced my examination but could not believe what I saw. The teeth were brilliant white in colour, but the gums were eroded and completely worn away, exposing the roots of the teeth. No wonder they were sensitive. I thought.

"Can I ask what toothpaste you use?" I enquired, searching for a clue.

"Ah Doc, I always use Vim." (Scouring powder, containing concentrated bleach.)

"May I suggest you stop using it, because it has corroded your gums as well as bleaching the teeth beyond belief."

"No way," he replied. There were no cameras in those days and no mobile phones to record this once in a career occurrence.

Here I was in my early twenties and learning fast. My nurse came in and told me my next patient was here, and although I hadn't seen her before, she had requested an extended appointment. She also said there was no way she was leaving me alone with this patient. Nicole came in, five feet ten inches, and with a figure that even the nurses admired.

"Mr Lester," she said and started to cry, "please mend my front teeth." This lady had been on a very poor diet combined with various recreational drugs, and the effect on her teeth was catastrophic. She would not smile because this showed dark brown cavities on all her front upper teeth. Cosmetically it was beyond poor and was obviously affecting her work and personal life. I went through the various options and we settled for crowns and bridges. This was not easy on the NHS, but gradually we restored her teeth and on her last visit she told me that she had just been accepted to work at the Playboy Club. She was absolutely delighted with the result and never stopped smiling. Such was the effect it had on her that the recommendations followed, and I had a constant stream of 'bunny girls' coming into the surgery, much to the suspicion of the staff. Later I heard that Nicole was enjoying a fruitful modelling job, and was drug free. (Triumph!)

Another memorable incident was when a mother came in with her daughter, who was to be married in six months. It was unusual for both to come into the surgery together, which in hindsight should have made me suspicious. The mother took the lead and said that she wanted her daughter to have full dentures before her wedding.

"Why?" I asked.

"So that she will look good on the photographs and have no further tooth problems." Incredible!

I examined the daughter and apart from a few cavities and a visit to the hygienist needed, she was in good shape. "She doesn't need full dentures and it would be criminal to make them for her," I said.

The daughter was very quiet but her mother replied, "I'm willing to pay privately for them." By this time, I was beginning to get annoyed but managed to keep my composure and stay cool.

"Madam, you don't understand. I won't make them because she doesn't need them, NHS or private."

Mother angry, and daughter embarrassed, they left the surgery with a parting shot. "I will go somewhere else then."

Sometimes ignorance is not bliss.

Chapter Nine
The Holistic Effect

Triumphs and disasters may come and go, but I want to tell you what it's really like to operate on patients, a simple filling or something more complex.

There is a constant palpable tension that emanates from almost every patient who enters the surgery, I can completely empathise with that. I know that with every injection for the patient there is a worry. Will it hurt? Will it numb the pain of the treatment? This anxious feeling is transmitted to the dentist, but from a different angle. Have I removed all the decay from a cavity? Does the filling look well and is the occlusion with opposing teeth correct? Will the patient be pleased or have any afterpain?

Dentistry is not just about the type of filling material used or if the colour match of a crown is perfect. Although these are important aspects of a treatment, I have always taken a more holistic approach to assessing a patient's needs, psychologically as well as orally. Remember the mouth is an extremely sensitive area and there is an almost intimate relationship between dentist and patient.

I have completed really excellent crowns and bridges, made dentures that have transformed the lives of elderly people, and ended pain for many patients. Of course, vitally important, but my treatment starts from the minute patients walk into my surgery. They have to feel genuinely welcome; I know they are nervous and this can make them sometimes ultra-defensive, so it is essential to put people at ease by talking about themselves before any dental issues. This means spending a few minutes just chatting. It could be about family, work, holidays, football or just their views on the world. I have always treated patients as if I was sitting in the dental chair; I would want to feel relaxed and interesting to the practitioner, and confident in their ability.

It does not finish when the patients have left the surgery. Often, after more invasive treatment, I would call to check and see how they were progressing and if any further issues had arisen. This was a genuine desire to demonstrate that dental care was ongoing and it was always greatly appreciated. I never considered aloofness to be an attribute in my career, and I have always endeavoured to go as far as possible to help those that have put trust in my professional abilities.

One particular episode demonstrates this philosophy. On a lovely family holiday in Crete, I received a telephone call from the surgery concerning a patient who was abroad and very concerned about her daughter, who had lost a filling and was having severe pain on eating and with cold fluids. I told my receptionist to ask the patient to call me, which she duly did. I thought at least I could give her some advice or direct her to a surgery.

"Where are you phoning from?" I asked.

Her reply amused me, "1`m in Crete." On enquiring where exactly on the island she was staying, I realised that she was within walking distance of my hotel. There were gasps of incredulity when I explained where I was. I then suggested she bring her daughter to the hotel. I delved into my emergency dental kit, a must-have when I am away, and a simple temporary dressing sorted the problem. A day later a bottle of wine was presented to us over dinner with compliments and many thanks for going out of my way to help. Triumph? Yes, but much more, I felt a great sense of wellbeing and contentment with my chosen profession.

Chapter Ten
Domiciliaries: The Good, the Bad and the Sad

Geriatric dentistry is most demanding, as patients are often confused and alone. Dentally, these patients are usually a neglected section of the population. I, with my staff, went to more than fifty residential care homes, some good, some bad and others just very sad places

The Good

You could tell the good ones immediately. The residents were clean and well looked after, the staff were interested in the wellbeing of the people in their care, and there were always children and grandchildren visiting. These places were uplifting. Dentistry was always going to be challenging in these circumstances, but in the main we managed oral health checks and made occasional dentures. This was always appreciated by the staff and relatives of the patients.

On one occasion, I went to a large residential home and asked to see Mrs H, who was ninety-two years old. "I'm sorry," was the reply, "you can't at the moment, she always goes to bed in the afternoon with Mr B, a new resident."

"Well, how long will she be?" I asked.

"At least an hour." I left impressed and returned later with all due respect.

Amidst all the difficulties there were some lighter moments. As I was seeing to an elderly gentleman, I bent down to pick up a box of gloves. Suddenly I felt by bottom being pinched and stroked. I turned around to see a lovely old lady smiling as she said, "Eh! You've got a bum just like my dear hubby used to have." Much laughter from the nursing staff. Apparently, she had a habit of doing this. (Triumph?)

As a matter of urgency, I was asked to see a new patient, who was losing weight and had no teeth. I arrived at the home with my nurse and my domiciliary bag which held all the instruments and materials I needed. We were shown into a smart clean bedroom where a frail lady was sitting in a chair. "Please make me some teeth," she begged. Apparently, she had no relatives and never received any visitors. I started with a full oral examination and found a large fungating mass in the mandible, (a type of lesion marked by ulcerations and tissue decay, common in advanced cases of cancer.) No question in my mind what this was. I told the staff to refer her to hospital immediately, which they duly did. Lo and behold, six months later and after surgery, I was asked to see her again. She looked well and animated and over the course of a few weeks we completed her new teeth. What a difference this made. She was delighted and we felt more than pleased, knowing we had given her a new lease of life. I continued to review her for many years, and the last time I saw her she was playing the piano in the lounge for the residents with a sparkling smile. (Triumph.)

The Bad

My nurse and I arrived at a new home in the suburbs of Manchester. As we went in, the smell of stale urine was pervading, the rooms were dirty and the residents looked lethargic and wandered about aimlessly. We looked around at the poor souls in the lounge, a few stale biscuits on the table and a fruit bowl with the fruit covered in flies. No relatives, no children and nobody seemed to care. We were taken to see a patient in a large bathroom and as we entered there was a person sitting on a commode.

"No," I said, "we are not seeing anyone in here." Then the strangest thing happened. A budgie flew around the room and landed in the hair of my nurse, where it deposited what remained of its digested lunch. After the hysterics from my nurse and we had cleaned up the mess, the said bird then landed on my bald pate, a much better place to sit. Enough! We left, sadly, never to return. (Disaster.)

I have been in care homes where there was human excrement on the floor and wet patches on chairs. I have seen food plates left on tables with no one attempting to clean up. I have seen staff sitting smoking and joking whilst residents just wandered about aimlessly. This was soul destroying and I cannot think of worse places to incarcerate people.

On one occasion we arrived at a new care home that we had not visited before. I rang the bell of what appeared to be a respectable place and the door was eventually opened by a large female resident who tried to push past us. Lying on the floor was a distressed diminutive nurse who had attempted to stop her from leaving. She was very upset and pleaded with us to stop the resident from leaving. With help from other staff members, we managed to restrain her, but not before I took a right hook to my jaw! Five minutes later she was calm and smiling. I had a bruise but was thanked for my efforts. I cannot possibly describe my innermost feelings following this incident. Using force to restrain a person who was obviously very confused is not part of my job description.

The Sad

Because you are old, or very old, does not preclude you from having dental treatment. It can be impossible to do many items of routine treatment, and often we had to refer to the local hospital. But we soldiered on, just looking and talking to these residents, listening to their stories and experiences. This seemed to help. But there were so many sad places where there was no stimulation, nor people to visit. These were the homes that left us feeling down.

On a domiciliary I was called to see an alcoholic man who was having difficulty eating. As I entered his house, the heat and alcohol smell was almost overpowering. After an examination, I explained that he needed a denture, that is an artificial removable plate with teeth added, on his lower jaw. We duly completed the treatment and on the final visit I asked him how often he was able to leave the house. His reply was staggering. "My two bottles of vodka are delivered each day, together with any food, so I haven't been out of my house for five years." After speaking to his GP, I realised there was nothing more that I could do to help. (Disaster.)

But Finally...

We were invited to many of the Christmas parties at the care homes, usually sumptuous affairs, and on these occasions the residents in their festive attire with paper hats genuinely seemed to be having fun and enjoying themselves.

Of all the stories to be told, there is one that will stay with me forever. We visited a lovely home quite near where I live and one of the residents, a Dr Elsie Begg, was quite lucid and in her nineties. When I saw her, she was dentally fit and was in good health.

"Dr Begg," I said, "you won't remember me, but you were my GP when I was a child. Not only that, you were the doctor who delivered me." She smiled as if searching for a distant memory. (Triumph.)

Chapter Eleven
The Private Surgery

My wife was pregnant with our first child in 1973 and we had to go and see an obstetrician in his rooms at St John Street, Manchester's Harley Street. Going into this beautiful Georgian building was surreal. "What a place for a surgery," I said to Sue. Three months later a mutual friend told me that a dentist in the same building in St John Street was due to retire and wanted somebody to take over; he was seventy-nine. That's when I met Alan and we got on famously. We agreed that I should take over, part time at first, until he was ready to leave. The surgery was very old fashioned with furniture that would horrify the Care Quality Commission today, but I knew it would be just perfect and so in 1975 I took over. See picture.

More than a little apprehensive, I arrived on my first day wearing a three-piece suit to look the part. I was about to work alongside some of the most eminent consultants in Manchester. (Triumph.) To say I felt out of my depth initially was correct; however, although I struggled and juggled with both surgeries and the domiciliaries, I gained in confidence, building up the practice over the next few years. Beverley joined me as my manageress and nurse, and is still with me after more than forty years. Most of the consultants and staff became patients and I became one part of the St John Street Medical Association.

Working here enabled me to complete more rarefied treatments. I made bridges for people who could not tolerate dentures, crowns and veneers and later implants. I was able to treat patients with no financial restrictions but I never gave up the NHS. Indeed, the NHS surgery was always the place where I could really feel that I was needed more, and so I divided my time between the two surgeries and considered that I had the best of both worlds. We re-equipped to give the place a more modern look, a new chair, new décor and a digital X-ray system. This was light years ahead of the equipment I had trained on. I had another trusted technician, Ray, who beavered away upstairs until he emigrated to Australia after many years.

Sam, a highly regarded consultant, was the chairman of the association and wanted to retire from that position. At a directors' meeting, he delivered his announcement about his choice of successor. "It has got to be Bernard Lester. He's here more than anybody else, is totally capable and is the logical choice." So, I was elected chairman of the most prestigious medical rooms in Manchester, and with the help of eminent consultant,

Roger Williams, the secretary, we managed the rooms until we sold the premises many years later. (Triumph.)

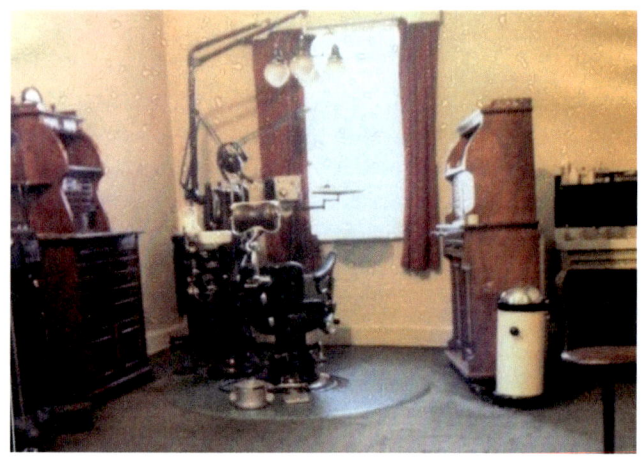

My private surgery, 1975

Chapter Twelve
The Actor, the Singer and the Radio Presenter

The Actor

A well-known Shakespearean actor was performing at the Opera House across the road from the private surgery. He came in complaining of toothache and said it was affecting his performances. I took a full history and X-rays and then the conversation went as follows.

Me: You have an old gold crown at the back lower and it has a vertical fracture of the root.

Him: Ah, all that glisters is not gold.

We agreed that an extraction was needed and it was to be completed straight away. My nurse prepared the local anaesthetic.

Me: I am going to give you a local anaesthetic now.

Him: Is this a dagger I see before me, the handle towards my hand?

I gave a local anaesthetic and we waited a few minutes before I explained that I was about to extract the tooth.

Him: Cowards die many times before their death, the valiant never taste of death but once.

Me: There we are, out in two pieces. We'll just stop the bleeding.

Him: (with a swab in his mouth) If you prick us do we not bleed? Lord what fools these mortals be!

Me: I have printed out a list of post-operative instructions for you, please read them.

Him: We have seen better days, but for my own part it was Greek to me.

Me: Neither a borrower nor a lender be. Here is your account!

I never saw him again as a patient, but I often did see him in various television dramas.

The Singer

SH was due to appear in the musical *Jesus Christ Superstar*; she was in the chorus but had been asked to understudy the main singers. She came to me in a terrible state as she had just been in a road traffic accident and had badly fractured her front incisor and the small adjacent lateral incisor. After examination and assessment of the damage, it was clear that there were root fractures and a lot of mobility of these two teeth; extraction was the only option. The teeth on either side, although heavily restored, were unaffected by the crash.

We planned to take the two teeth out and I made what we call an immediate denture that fits over the extractions straight away, so at least she would look better. The problem was, her singing, with a denture on her palate, would be affected. She was warned about this but we had no option. The teeth were painful and infected. The extractions were uneventful and we fitted the partial denture, which greatly improved her appearance, but she was lisping badly and very upset.

We only had ten weeks before she was due to start rehearsals, so with this in mind we had a meeting with the patient and my technicians. Because the teeth on either side of the gap were heavily filled, we decided to crown these two teeth and build a bridge across. This was a fairly routine job but the difficulty was making sure that the diction was perfect. We had a model of how the teeth were after the accident and photographs so that we could copy the position as near as possible. The preparations were done, impressions taken and temporary crowns fitted. Then a week later she came in to have the bridge fitted.

Now for this appointment we had two technicians ready to do any alterations needed, together with the patient's partner and singing coach to give advice. We removed the temporary crowns and fitted the bridge with a loose temporary cement and showed the patient.

"Wow," she said," it's better than before and looks perfect."

"We need to test the diction," said the coach, and produced a song sheet for *Jesus Christ Superstar*. Without a second thought and with a most beautiful voice, she began to sing the main song. We were all stunned and impressed by the power of her voice.

"No," complained the coach. "There's still a slight lisp."

We took the bridge off three times for alterations, and only when the coach was completely satisfied, did we cement the bridge in position. She was delighted and as we opened the surgery door, we were given a full rendition of *I don't know how to love him*. From the waiting room I could hear applause and a shout of 'more' from the reception.

A week later an envelope arrived with four tickets to watch her perform. (Triumph!)

The Radio Presenter

"Bernard, an urgent phone call for you from BBC Radio in Manchester," Bev said with a smile. This was it I thought, recognition at last, an interview, articles in the papers and television? No! They had one of their presenters with a dental problem. A strange conversation followed:

Me: Hello, what's the problem?

BBC: One of our star lady presenters is having some dental issues.

Me: And what is her problem?

BBC: I don't know. You're the dentist.

Me: Look I'm only asking what trouble she is having. (Increasingly exasperated)

BBC: How would I know!

Me: Please ask her.

BBC: I can't, she's on air at the moment.

Me: Pass her a note and ask her what the problem is.

BBC: That's a good idea.

I was left holding the phone for five minutes whilst the search was on for pen and paper I assumed.

BBC: She's lost a crown and needs it re-fixing.

Me: I can see her at my surgery, three p.m. this afternoon.

BBC: What! Can't you come here and do it?

Me: No. Would she move out of her studio to do her programme?

BBC: Well, yes, she does often.

Me: Would you like me to move my dental chair and equipment to your studio? (Sarcasm)

BBC: Would you do that? Awfully good of you.

Me: No, I won't, I was being funny! Give her the appointment and tell her to get to the surgery, here.

The crown was recemented with no problems. Four months later I received payment. (Triumph.)

Chapter Thirteen
Dentist or Gynaecologist?

Our wonderful gynaecologist, in the private rooms, Geoffrey, was occasionally sending patients to see me to check their dental fitness. Often the patient would have consecutive appointments with the two of us. Mrs R came in as a new patient to see me, walked through my door, sat at my dental unit and announced without a word from me, "I think I'm pregnant, can you confirm this for me, as I would like to have any treatment completed as a private patient?"

After a slight hesitation from me and a gasp from the staff I responded, "But I am here to check your teeth."

"Oh my God!" she exclaimed." I have the two appointments mixed up".

Reception then phoned me to explain what had happened and the patient, suitably embarrassed, went to see the gynaecologist and came back an hour later to see me. Yes, she was pregnant. The patient remained with me for many years, together with the twins that she went on to give birth to.

Geoffrey delivered all my three children. The youngest, Rebecca, was born at a most inconvenient time, just when England were playing Germany in the World Cup. In between Sue`s contractions, we were dashing into the common room to see the match on TV, and Sue conveniently gave birth just after the game had ended. The match was goalless, but amidst much joviality, Sue was not pleased that our attention was somewhat distracted from the delivery room.

Now it's not often a dentist becomes involved with a delivery, but I was asked to see a pregnant patient of mine who was about to give birth. Geoffrey was in charge of the case but asked me to deal with the patient's dental discomfort in hospital. I saw her in the delivery suite and found that she had lost a filling which was causing her "More pain than the bloody baby." I put a temporary dressing in, which seemed to do the job for her, but just as I had finished, Geoffrey said, "The baby`s coming, push, please."

I did. I pushed off as quickly as I could.

Chapter Fourteen
Help is at Hand: The Associates

As the years rolled on my routine seemed set. I beavered away on the NHS and witnessed many changes in the way we were remunerated. From the start it was a pay per item service, which was not perfect but certainly had advantages over the units of dental activity system (UDA), which followed the original system. The idea was that you received UDAs according to treatments, and the dentist was awarded a certain number of these units depending on the historical turnover of the practice. This way the NHS could know precisely what the dental system would cost them and strangely we always struggled to make the target set by the government.

Associates are dentists who are either newly qualified or do not yet have their own surgeries, which is exactly how I started. The idea is that they gain experience in running a surgery and in treating patients that are given to them by the principal. My NHS surgery was now very busy as we worked in quite a deprived area. I'd had several associate dentists working for me, some good and some, in my opinion, bad.

The local health authority had been very helpful and funded a new surgery complete with a digital X-ray system, which meant we had the result in seconds. No more dark rooms with fixer and developer. This was a very generous decision by the authority and meant that we could increase the NHS capacity. Strangely we then received a call from the managers in charge of implementing the new UDA system, to say that they would not fund, with a UDA allowance, a dentist for the new surgery, which was standing pristine and unused. The associate due to start was excellent and raring to go, but we had no funds for him. I was furious that in this part of Manchester some bureaucrat was trying to squeeze a full service without allowing for any expansion of the surgery. When I told the department about the new dentist, the reply was, "Well, he will have to work somewhere else."

Okay, I thought, I need to speak to my MP, who was a Mancunian born and bred. He knew the district well and was astounded at the lack of intelligent thinking that had gone into the decision. "I will see what I can do," he promised.

Two weeks later I received a call from the bureaucrats to say the decision had been reversed, and they were going to fund the new dentist. (Triumph!)

The new associate stayed with me for many years and eventually took over from me.

Chapter Fifteen
The Kidnapping

A terrifying experience brought a long-standing patient to the surgery. She was in considerable distress. I had taken her on as a patient from my predecessor at my private rooms. I had seen her for many years and her husband was very well known in the financial world, and a knight of the realm. I had completed a front bridge for her to replace the denture, and she was thrilled, saying she could eat properly and bite into things normally. This was going to prove pivotal to what subsequently happened.

My treatment would make or break this patient's recovery, but this was an awful and unique case. As the wife of a prominent business man, she was identified by a villain as a valuable target, and was kidnapped and badly beaten, before being pushed into the boot of a car by a man who then attempted to blackmail her husband to effect her release. Her hands and feet were bound together with heavy cord, and sometime afterwards, she told me that she had expected to die in that position. With amazing determination and a cool head, she managed somehow to bite through the bonds using her new front bridge, releasing her hands then her feet. She crawled out of the boot of the vehicle when it stopped. The car was parked in a side street but, although it was dark, she managed to crawl along the pavement until a passing motorist stopped. The police and ambulance were called. This sounds more like an unlikely TV drama, but it really did happen.

The first I knew about it was when I read the story in the *Manchester Evening News*, where it was headlined. The criminal was eventually apprehended and convicted.

Three weeks later her husband called me and I was asked to go to the hospital to see her, but I was warned that he thought the damage to her teeth was irreversible, since she had been hit with a baseball bat. As I entered the hospital, there were journalists from the national press interviewing him. I quietly bypassed them and went up to see my patient. I did not recognise her; such was the extent of her facial injuries. I sat at her bedside and took notes of the damage, promising I would do my very best to restore her appearance and teeth. The problem was not just physical; it was the profound psychological effect the incident had on this once very confident and striking woman.

After a fortnight she came into the surgery for X-rays and photographs. I sat down with them both, outlining the options and my treatment plan. She looked grey and gaunt, not the vibrant and confident woman that I knew. I worried then that this would be a defining treatment for her, and probably for me.

The procedure took three months, during which time she needed the recently completed upper bridge replaced together with numerous crowns and other bridge replacements. The damage had been horrific, but the strength of the bridges had protected the roots of her teeth. Amazingly, no extractions were needed.

As the treatment progressed, we could see a gradual improvement. On completion, the patient and her husband thanked me and left, but we felt utterly deflated. We thought there would be some sort of fanfare at the end of this challenging case.

Then, a few days later we received a letter from her husband and I have copied it verbatim.

Dear Mr Lester,

I am very pleased indeed with the result which has been achieved. More importantly, however, my wife is delighted with the result, and this has done more than any other single thing to restore her confidence, and get into the frame of mind where she is now prepared to face the world again, and take up life where we left off three months ago. This is something which is beyond price, and we are both very grateful indeed for your inestimable help in this direction.

Yours sincerely...

(Triumph.)

We then had a call from his secretary saying that she was back to her normal self and everybody was delighted. (Definitely Triumph!)

Later in the year, I was wined and dined at the Midland Hotel by the two of them, and it was an absolute pleasure to see her restored and shining again.

After this case I developed a habit of sitting in my office after surgery, allowing all the invasive procedures I had completed to be filtered and contemplated. Yes, I had done my day's work, but had I made mistakes? Could I have done better for the patients? Would they be happy with my treatment? This was akin to switching a computer off, which it probably was. (Sometimes Triumph, sometimes Disaster.)

Chapter Sixteen
The Smoker, the Stripper, the Pheasant… and the Lost Lunch

The Smoker

Mr H, high up in a multinational company, came in to see me with a strange complaint. He'd had an upper premolar extracted whilst abroad, six weeks prior to his visit to see me. He was a heavy smoker, and complained of not being able to suck properly on a cigarette. Also, when drinking, he felt that fluid was going into the back of his nose. Ah, I thought, this is a rare event and sounds like an oroantral fistula. What can occasionally happen after an extraction is that an opening is made into the sinus of the upper jaw. Now the sinus is connected to the nose via the ostia, which means he could not draw properly on a cigarette and fluids would go from his mouth to the back of his nasal cavities.

So, as he put it, "Smoking a ciggy takes me bloody ages." I asked him to hold his nostrils closed and blow to raise the pressure in them. Sure enough, there was the tell-tale stream of bubbles and air from where the tooth had been extracted. Eureka! I confirmed the diagnosis with an X-ray and gave him the option of a referral to the dental hospital, or I could seal it for him. I explained that I knew the theory, but I had never attempted the procedure before.

"You do it, Doc, I'm not going to a bleeding hospital."

He came in for his surgery and I was suitably gowned up with all my new and unused surgical instruments ready and waiting. I gave a local anaesthetic, lifted a small flap of the mucous membrane and stitched it closed. I then fitted an acrylic splint to keep it covered and told him not to blow his nose until his next appointment.

He came back to see me six weeks later, walked into the surgery and promptly lit a cigarette:

"Magic, Doc, I can smoke a ciggy properly now." He continued smoking whilst he told me how he was trying to stop and had reduced to thirty a day already.

I can't decide whether that goes down as a successful case or not.

The Stripper

I am now the proud owner of a black belt in free style karate, with a certificate on show next to my other degrees. Ms P came in for a routine examination as a private patient. She was an attractive lady, early thirties, with an alluring and mischievous smile, married twice and now working as an 'exotic dancer'. During the treatment, I could see her looking at my new karate certificate and photograph on the wall, and every few minutes she would look at it again.

After we had finished, she asked me if she could borrow a karate outfit, known as a GI, for her act. "Of course, I will be glad to help. I have an old outfit you can use."

Ms P was delighted, and yet I felt something disturbing but could not put my finger on it. "I will bring you some photographs when I can," she promised, on her way out of the surgery.

One month later a brown paper envelope was posted through the main door to the building and it was opened without a thought by my manageress, Bev, in front of the downstairs receptionists, and the rest of my staff. There was a sudden gasp then laughter from everyone and fingers pointing.

"Dr Lester, what have you been up to?" exclaimed Bev. I looked at the photographs and there was Ms P, wearing my karate outfit, with her ample breasts on full display and in various poses.

"Oh, what lovely photographs," I muttered sheepishly.

"What about your name on the front of the outfit where everyone can see, that's some advertisement for you," Bev said.

What? I sank slowly into my chair and tried to disappear. (Disaster?)

The Pheasant

Mr S came in on an emergency appointment, a lovely gentleman who had been a patient for some considerable time. He was a hunter fisherman type with wonderful stories to tell. On this occasion he had returned from a shooting event the night before, but when he started to eat, he found that he was not able to close his teeth together. He said they'd had a pheasant dinner the night of the shoot, but then after was in a considerable amount of pain.

My brain cells were already putting pieces of the jigsaw together and I asked him if they had eaten one of the pheasants that had been recently shot? It turned out that it was, but it had been hanging for some time. I examined him and found a piece of lead shot from the shotgun cartridge neatly wedged into the filling. This was removed with a minimum of effort and the patient went out smiling. Revenge of the pheasant, I think. See below.

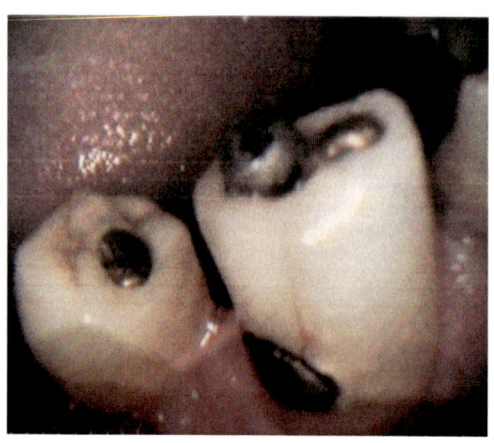

Spot the lead shot

The Lost Lunch

Mrs D was a lovely vivacious and very sensitive lady who owned one of the best Spanish restaurants in Manchester. Whenever she came to see us, she insisted on taking the last appointment of the morning so that, as she put it, "I can bring you all a little flavour of Spain for your lunch." Naturally her visits were always eagerly anticipated, and the wonderful Spanish omelette she brought in with a delicious crisp salad was devoured with relish by all the staff.

It was a glorious spring morning, with the sun beaming into the surgery, made better when we realised Mrs D had taken her usual appointment, the last of the session. "No need to go out for sandwiches today," I told Bev.

But Mrs D arrived in the surgery in floods of tears and inconsolable. We settled her down and asked what had happened to make her so upset. "I've left your omelette and salad and some special cakes on the bus on the empty seat that was next to me, and I only realised when I arrived at the surgery."

"Don't worry," said Bev, "I'll phone the bus company to see if it's been found."

No lost packages were located on any of the buses on that route, and so we explained to Mrs D that it was simply unfortunate, not to be concerned, and then made her a further appointment. Although still visibly upset, she insisted on going straight home.

Bev set off to the local supermarket and collected sandwiches. (Disaster.)

An hour into the afternoon session Mrs D phoned the surgery. "You will not believe what happened," she exclaimed in excitement. "I caught my usual bus home and by coincidence sat in the same seat as I did on my way to the surgery. I could not believe my eyes! There was the omelette, salad and cakes exactly where I'd left them this morning." What did she do with our lunch? "I gave it all to the driver of the bus," she told us. "He was really pleased."

I bet he was, I mused. (Disaster again!)

Chapter Seventeen
Dentistry and the Law

My friend, Gary, had been busy with his own surgeries but then decided to complete a legal course in order to see negligence and personal injury cases. He invited me to join him in this new project and to date we have now been working together for twenty-five years. There is a huge chasm between the serious cases, some involving awful abuse, for instance where staff at one residence extracted a loose tooth with a fork on an unfortunate individual, and some of the much simpler accident cases.

Of the serious cases, I am not willing to divulge further details. Some of the negligence ones are in areas where any dentist could be involved. Dentists are human so mistakes can be made. In others cases, in my opinion, it is plain to see that the patient can only see a pound sterling sign.

The personal injury cases are usually because of road traffic accidents, or sometimes just unfortunate occurrences. On one occasion, a young girl came to see us with a broken molar which fractured on a chip. We asked what happened and she replied that she bit into the chip and heard a crack. We asked what was inside the item to cause this damage. She then produced a two-inch screw which had fallen out from the top of the range at the chip shop, into the deep fat fryer together with the other chips. Fractured tooth and an implant needed.

Then the case of the nut, without the screw, which nestled nicely in a pizza. The unfortunate patient bit down on it and smashed a front tooth. Root treatment and post crown needed. These are some of the cases we have seen, but others can be much more serious and the damage caused extensive. Some of these accidents happened at school with the child involved in sport. It is important to note that in law, the patient must have their teeth restored to the condition they were in before the accident, if possible. This may involve ongoing expenses for replacement at various intervals; a crown for example, would need to be replaced every ten to twelve years.

On one occasion we were asked by a solicitor to see an inmate at the local prison. Apparently, he had severe toothache and bought some cocaine to kill the pain, which may well have worked. Unfortunately, it was a kilo that he had purchased, which was difficult to explain.

I can honestly say that I have learnt much from some of the negligence cases that I have seen, and several times I've seen cases where the wrong tooth has been extracted. There is no defence against this and often the cost of rectifying the situation can be high. I now always do a double check as well as confirming with the patient which tooth is the culprit.

Chapter Eighteen
The Story So Far

I was now the proud father of three children, growing up fast. None were interested in dentistry, and my son, Andrew, would not even talk about the possibility. He told me that the thought of putting cotton wool in a patient's mouth made him nauseous. We had extended the house to accommodate the children and so life was hectic with schools, examinations and all the lovely day to day routines that we will look back on in our dotage. My father-in-law died, and this had a profound effect on me as it was the first time that I had to face up to mortality. Some years later my own father died in hospital and although I knew he was not in the best of health, it was a terrible shock. I was on a domiciliary visit on a Sunday when I got the call that he had collapsed, and I do not remember driving to the hospital. I can recall now, as a child, the first time he took me to the Manchester Microscopic Society meeting and persuaded me to look at my own blood on a slide. I can still remember the sharp stab on my thumb as a sample was taken and the pride in taking the slide home with me.

Both surgeries were busy, and so I decided that I would like to do a further degree course, the Member of the Joint Dental Faculty (MJDF). I relished this new academic challenge. There were so many more aspects of dentistry to learn, and I completed two years of study before taking my final exam. Back to being a student again and I loved it. The examinations were to be taken at the prestigious Royal College of Surgeons in London. It was just like finals again, written papers, spotters, and there were cubicles with a description of the patient inside and their symptoms, with actors playing various parts. Now it had been a long day and I was on my last cubicle, a case of mouth ulcers. I was probably the oldest person taking the exam and the most experienced. I walked into the room and was confronted by a very glamorous actress who seemed very upset with herself, and an external examiner who was not in the mood, after a long session, to take prisoners. The conversation went as follows.

Me: Good afternoon. What's the problem?

Actress: I have the most terrible mouth ulcers, I get them regularly.

Me: One alone or do they seem to come in crops?

Actress: Oh, hundreds at a time.

Me: Mm, how is this condition affecting you?

Actress: I can't eat salty foods and wine irritates my mouth. I have difficulty kissing my partner and it's affected him so much that he walked out on me yesterday.

Me: Do you have ulcers anywhere else?

Actress: I beg your pardon. I do not like what you are inferring!

At this stage I detected a slight smile from her and a snigger from the external examiner. I'm winning!

Actress: They are just in my mouth.

Me: How long have you had them?

Actress: About five days.

Me: Do you smoke?

Actress: No. Why do you ask?

Me: Because they may be more common in non-smokers, one of the few things that is. When do these ulcers appear?

Actress: At least once a month.

Me: Are you taking the birth control pill?

Actress (flustered): Why what makes you ask that?

Me: There is a report that says there may be a connection.

Actress: We are trying for a baby, or were before he walked out on me.

Me: I recommend an antiseptic mouthwash to start with, and I would like you to keep a diary of when you get ulcers. We can try you on some topical steroids and refer you to a specialist if they persist for more than three weeks at a time. That's all for now.

External: Are you sure? You have another three minutes for further questions.

He took a glass of water.

Sometimes I feel mischievous and want to be silly or controversial, I'm not sure which. So, I came up with another question.

Me: Would you like to join me for a drink and a chat afterwards?

External, spluttering his water: That will not get you any extra marks!

Actress with a smile that said 'that was fun': I can't, the alcohol hurts the ulcers."

We all laughed and I bid the two of them a good evening.

The next day I was notified that I had passed. I now hold the degree MJDF RCS. (Triumph.)

Then I received the final invoice for the course. (Disaster.)

Chapter Nineteen
Age Creeping Up

It was 2006, and I had a shock. A letter from the NHS pension people arrived informing me that my pension was due on my sixtieth birthday in January the following year. This came as a real jolt because the word pension I always thought spelt the beginning of the end of my life. A week or two later, my associate and I were having dinner and a chat discussing the various problems we had, both personal and professional. Out of the blue he asked me if I was thinking of selling the NHS practice. This was not a complete surprise because we had discussed my possible next move after my trauma of the pension letter.

"That's fine," I said, surprising myself. We agreed on all the issues there and then and that I was to continue working for him as an associate. Done and dusted, the surgery would continue in good hands.

My sixtieth birthday came along together with my pension but the day after, my dear mother died. Suddenly myself and two brothers were alone without our parents. Although we had all looked after her, I often wished I would have taken more time out to see her. Hindsight can be corrosive and disturbing by opening up darker chasms in your life.

The private practice was now very busy and I was enjoying the clinical work and the wonderful people I worked with. Originally, we owned two buildings in St. John Street with shared common connecting areas, but age was wearing us down in numbers a little, together with the deaths of our wonderful gynaecologist and ear, nose and throat specialists.

Running such big houses was very expensive and we had in the previous five years renovated both premises at quite a cost. It was at this point as we were looking through the rooms, that I found a very dull pencil sketch with the name L S Lowry at the bottom. Quite a find, and I often wonder why it took us so long to recognise it. We had it valued and it was bought by one of the doctors in our house.

So we sold one half of the property and all moved into the building where my surgery was located. This proved to be a cost-effective move as well as fully utilising the space we had available. The people who moved in next door now also represented aspects of health management and was run by doctors.

On the day of the completion, we all worked hard in emptying the sold premises, and as I recall it was a very warm day. The very last item to be moved was a very heavy examination chair, and I have a wonderful memory of the board's secretary, Roger, sitting in the chair in the car park in the sun, where he fell asleep. We left him there a little while to recover.

The funds had helped us, but it was becoming apparent that as our association was reducing in numbers, the income from tenants was reducing. The die had been cast and the sun was setting on our wonderful St. John Street Medical Association. When the people who had purchased our next-door building asked us if we wished to sell the second property and remain as tenants, we had our last monthly meeting and accepted their offer.

We had our last Christmas party at the rooms and we were all there to give speeches, and sit around drinking champagne, when suddenly the door opened from one of the consulting rooms and out popped a patient who had been seeing one of our neurologists. We all forgot that he was still working, and I will never forget his words when he saw us sitting on the stairs in a jolly but reflective mood, drinks in hand, canapés on the tables, laughing and reminiscing.

"Blimey, I've never seen a surgery like this. I'm coming back here again." As he was the last patient to be seen before we became tenants, we gave him a glass of champagne, and he was delighted.

Chapter Twenty
Such Wonderful Staff

What can I say about the people who have worked for me for virtually the whole of my career? I have been truly blessed with the most wonderful staff who have helped run the surgeries and guided me through good times and bad. I have been through five divorces (not mine!) with them, remarriages, children and grandchildren. They hardly ever took time off for sickness and only took basic maternity leave. My technicians have all been loyal to me and honest in their advice, and not afraid to criticise me when it was justified.

We shared more than a surgery; we shared a profession, a camaraderie and a friendship which has endured. We were like a family that shared the squabbles, the laughter and the sad times together, and even now we all try to meet up at reunions every few months. The patients loved us for the stability and convivial atmosphere; there was always a familiar face when they came into the surgery, and it was this bonding we had with them which set us apart. I had to give prizes at my old local primary school, and it was here that I met one of my old teachers, now retired, who put me in my place by saying with a smile, "I knew you wouldn't do much with your life." (Disaster!) None of us had moved more than a few miles from where we were born and I feel that we have all contributed significantly to the dental health of the area.

Now a lesson in how to keep your staff. Most have stayed with me all my professional life. Why? You may ask. Is it because I'm a super dentist with magnetic personality and oodles of charm? No, I am a good dentist who treated my staff as if they were an integral part of the surgery, which indeed they were. They each had a job to do and they were well paid for doing it. Not only this, there was maternity leave, time off when they had personal problems and holidays, and I always made sure that during the good and bad times, they were financially taken care of to the best of my ability. In return, they were loyal and always put the patients first. They were unstinting in their support for me and the work we did for our community.

We had many wonderful Christmas parties, for instance we would go to the Playboy Club, and strangely, I always received preferential treatment there. The Midland hotel and many other venues were places of choice. This was a time, after a heavy year, to relax and take stock. They were times for the staff to let their hair down, which was difficult for me because I didn't have much. We talked about who was pregnant, who was getting divorced, and any other gossip we could think of.

On one occasion we went to London for the day and had the most wonderful taxi driver who took us all round the main sites. We stopped at Windsor and while the girls were looking at the shops, Prince Charles casually came out of a famous shoe shop saying, "Good morning, ladies." That was it! They were convinced that I had friends at the palace and had arranged it all for them. "A few phone calls did it," I said casually.

Sometimes you have to repay loyalty. My NHS manageress, Susan, who hardly ever had a day off, talked constantly about seeing Michelangelo's *David* at the Accademia in Florence. She would look at pictures and complain that she would never get the chance to see it for real. Secretly I made enquiries about the possibility of a trip to Florence for the day.

"We're not having a Christmas party in December this year, I thought we would go in January instead."

Groans in response and a chorus of, "Well, where will we go?"

My enigmatic reply was, "I'll find a nice Italian restaurant somewhere".

I had now booked for us all to go to Florence, seven a.m. flight out and back the same day at nine-thirty p.m. A few weeks before the trip, I called the staff together: "Make sure your passports are up to date. That Italian meal we are going to have is in Florence."

There were squeals of excitement and typical gasps of, "Oh my God, what am I going to wear?"

Well, we made it to the airport and after a two-hour flight we landed at Pisa airport, where we boarded a coach to Florence. "Hello, Mr Lester, fancy seeing you all here," said two patients who were on the flight. We still talk about the coincidence with them whenever they are in the surgery. Taxi to the Accademia and there it was. The most magnificent sculpture of *David*. There were plenty of tears, but we then had our authentic Italian lunch and wandered around Florence, spotting all the landmarks from the film *Hannibal*. We were back on time and, after a day to remember, made our way home. (Triumph).

Not too long after the trip, one of my nurses became very ill and tragically died. This was more than a shock; it was like losing a close family member. The funeral was the saddest affair, and to this day we still keep photographs of her in the surgery.

Chapter Twenty-One
Successes

What a surprise, we entered a competition and won!

Wow! In the competition you had to state the reasons for your surgery's success. I made the point that what was most important was all the people who worked there with me. The judges seemed to agree and rewarded us with six bottles of champagne. (Triumph!)

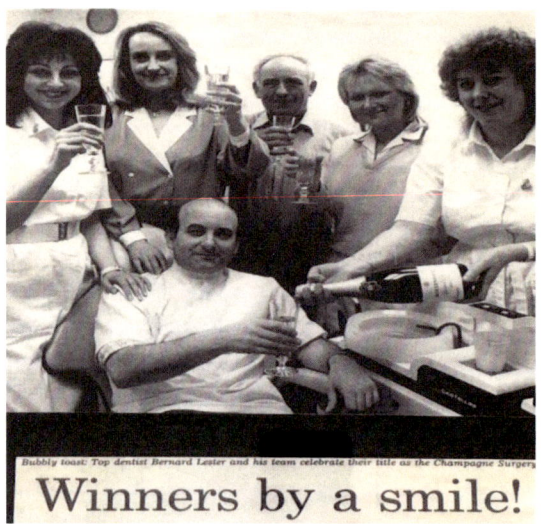

Bubbly toast: Top dentist Bernard Lester and his team celebrate their title as the Champagne Surgery

Winners by a smile!

Kind permission of the Manchester Evening News

I don't think I can say that I've saved a life in my clinical career, although I may have come close. I have, however, certainly influenced many lives.

Mrs P had been coming to see me for many years and on this day, she came into the surgery for a routine examination. I thought that she looked rather pale but continued with the examination. When I looked at her eyes, I thought she appeared a little anaemic. After we had finished, I advised her, "Look, I'm not sure, but I think you may be slightly anaemic. Can you see your GP for a blood test?"

A week later she called me to tell me that she had followed my advice and asked for a blood test with her GP. Her doctor told her it was not needed, but Mrs P insisted and a sample was taken. Twenty- four hours later she received an urgent call from them to return to the surgery as soon as possible. She was told that her iron and haemoglobin levels were dangerously low. She was admitted to hospital where they found a small ulceration of the bowel that was bleeding, caused by the medication she was taking for an existing condition. In another few weeks she would have needed major surgery for a perforation. I received a letter from the patient saying that she was so delighted with the care I had taken with my examination and recommendation to see her GP. She was now on iron supplements and had made a full recovery.

As I explained earlier, a bridge in dentistry is where teeth are crowned and used as supports for extra teeth to fill gaps in the mouth. Sometimes these spaces can be small, maybe two or three units, a unit being a space or a tooth; others can be long span bridges with many gaps to fill and teeth to crown to support. Ideally the teeth to be crowned already have fillings in them or other restorations. In the late seventies, Ms T came in wearing an upper denture which was unsatisfactory, causing her awful speech problems. Her confidence was low and she was visibly upset. There were no implants at that time, and I don't think they would have been of use for this patient. We decided that a long span bridge was the best option, twelve units, a full arch in other words. This was by far the largest bridge that I had done and so we left a full morning for the preparations. Two weeks later, and after a few try-in appointments, we were ready to finish. We showed the patient the result in the mirror and she was overjoyed. There were now no obvious speech difficulties so we cemented the bridge into position. In 2017 I received the following email.

Hello Bernard. Recently I read that a dental bridge has a life of 10-15 years. I thought you would like to know how your 'vintage' work was doing. In the mid-seventies you did a twelve-unit bridge for me, it transformed my life. After I moved, I found a new dentist who has since retired. I know the new one will be impressed by your work as has everyone who has had cause to see it. So not before time I'd like to say renewed thanks for a remarkable bit of dentistry. Not sure how much longer it will keep going but I've had 40-odd years of mentally thanking you almost every time I clean my teeth. (Triumph.)

Ms T.

The provision of implants is an aspect of dentistry that has made an important impact on treatment options. This was already filtering through into public consciousness so now patients were asking about the possibility as an alternative after extractions. With this in mind I went to London to complete the course at Nobel Pharma and came back confused. In the early days there were so many different components to assemble; it was a minefield. Together with a colleague, an oral surgeon, who worked in our private rooms, we mastered the rudiments.

Our first patient was a lovely lady called Margaret who, she claimed, was seventy-five years old and wearing a full upper denture. She was adamant that she needed an alternative as it was spoiling her quality of life, causing her embarrassment because they were always loose due to the anatomy involved. After examination, X-rays and scans, the surgeon put five implants in place with no issues. We then had to wait six months for the implants to fully integrate into the bone. They were then exposed so that I could complete the restoration. The final bridge was fitted and Margaret was absolutely delighted with the result, as were we. We saw her regularly for the next five years when she would always come in and say it was the best thing she had ever done, making an amazing difference to her life. Sadly, she died at the age we thought of eighty. Her friend came in to see me at a later date and as we talked about Margaret, we discovered that she was actually ninety when she died. She had told us she was ten years younger, presumably because she thought she may have been too old for implants. To be fair, we never suspected that there was any intentional deceit, and we assumed that the mistake was simply a communication error. Either way it made no difference to the final treatment, which was an all-round success. (Triumph.)

Chapter Twenty-Two
The Tooth, the Whole Tooth and Nothing but the Tooth

Occasionally, something happens in the surgery that touches you deeply. Usually it's a thank you card, or a phone call from a grateful patient, but on this occasion, it was completely different.

Master Jimmy, age seven, came into the surgery with his parents because he had a very loose upper front first tooth which was causing him problems. The tooth would have come out by itself in a few days and was hanging by a thread. I decided to extract it and so we put in a small amount of anaesthetic and I explained to him that I would use my fingers to take out the little remaining piece of tooth.

"That's okay, but can I have the tooth back so the fairies will pay me for it?"

"Of course," I said as I confidently pulled the tooth out between my fingers. "The Chinese method," I proudly exclaimed, at which point the tooth slid out of my fingers into the crease of the chair and disappeared. Jimmy was distraught, not because of the extraction, but because he had lost the money from the fairies. We all tried our best to console him but to no avail. We could not find the tooth, and I could see that the boy was not going to leave the surgery until we had succeeded in finding it. There was no choice but to dismantle the dental chair and search for it. I removed the seat and tried to move the wires that fed the electric mechanism. Bingo! I spotted the renegade tooth next to an electrical junction, but how to retrieve it? No choice, I picked my finest narrow root forceps, which maybe I should have used in the first place, and grabbed the tooth, but out it popped again.

"This tooth does not want to come out," I sighed. A different instrument had to be called upon, one of my long Spencer Wells, which is now in my fishing box (very useful). "Got it!" I shouted, to cheers from all present. Jimmy was ecstatic, so we carefully washed it and put it into a special box. "How much will the fairies give you?" I asked.

"One pound I think." We were all delighted with the outcome, and I spent the next hour trying to put the dental unit back together.

About a week later, I received an envelope and a note from Jimmy in his own writing. Inside was a fifty pence piece taped to the note which read, "Thank you, Bernard, for finding my tooth and because you went to so much trouble, I want to share the money from the fairies."

I was lost for words, and very touched by such a thoughtful gesture. I wanted to return it but how?

Bev came up with the idea of sending a letter back, from the fairies, with two shiny new one-pound coins inside, saying how impressed they were with his generosity.

Sometimes children can be the most difficult patients, or just amazing, and in particular there are two cases that confirm how challenging they can be in the surgery.

Firstly, Mrs H came in with her eight-year-old son for a first visit, and after the preliminaries, I saw that there was one early filling to be completed in a remaining first tooth. It was decided that a local anaesthetic was not needed as the cavity was very shallow. Whilst I was explaining to mum the procedure, the child hot-footed it out of the surgery and through the front door, much to his mother's distress. I dashed out after him, together with my nurse, the receptionist and the child's mother. The 'fab four' caught up with him in the park a few hundred yards from the surgery, where we found him hiding in some bushes. The sight of some gowned-up people chasing after a boy seemed to alert the local passers-by, who looked on with amusement. Eventually we persuaded him back into the surgery, but after our exertions we decided to rebook the appointment. (Disaster.) However, we did see him again and he remained a patient for many years after and we, to his embarrassment, always called him our runaway. (Triumph.)

The second memorable case was a quite unruly child who insisted on kicking his mother, who was trying her best to placate him. I decided to intervene, gently restraining him, whilst politely asking him to stop. We managed to complete the treatment, and the mother was very grateful. On her way out her comment that her child "Respects discipline" left me stunned, and this idea that the use of physical force was in some way to be commended made me vow never in any way to try to restrain a patient, no matter the circumstances. (Disaster.)

Chapter Twenty-Three
The Snorer

Wendy came into the surgery as a new patient, very genuinely upset and complaining of snoring every night, to such an extent that her new husband would not sleep in the same bedroom. This was obviously causing her great distress, and I dare say her husband as well. After completing a full examination, we discussed the treatment options, and decided to construct an anti-snoring appliance. This works on the principle that if the lower jaw is set in a protrusive position overnight, the snoring will be reduced or stopped, in theory. It was not difficult to fit once the appliance was made, and after giving the patient instructions for use, we told her to call or make an appointment in three weeks.

It was actually two weeks later that she called and the conversation was, shall we say, enlightening:

Wendy: Mr Lester, it worked. You have stopped me snoring.

Me: Oh good, are you having any difficulty using it?

Wendy: No, I always take it out when we make love.

Me : Oh! That's erm good isn't it?

Wendy: It's marvellous. You know last night because I wasn't snoring, he slept with me. Well, I can tell you it was a night to remember! After the third time...

Cutting her conversation short...

Me: Oh, I'm really pleased, Wendy. Shall I see you for your routine examination?

Wendy: Yes, please, and my husband wants to come in also. And by the way, thank you for saving my love life, and marriage.

Too much detail I think, but there you go, now I'm a sex therapist. (Triumph.)

A week later I received a call from the local radio station, asking me to give an interview about the snoring appliance. It seemed Wendy had contacts with them. The interview was going smoothly with my most professional voice until the radio presenter suggested, "It's a bit of a passion killer, isn't it?"

Ah, I thought, I know where this is coming from.

"Well," I said, "you can always take it out if it is likely to interfere with anything planned."

So that's covered some memorable successes. But, Bernard, do not get carried away. See the next chapter...

Chapter Twenty-Four
The Failures

A letter arrived marked private and confidential, with the name of a solicitor stamped on it. Ominous. This has probably happened to every dentist. It usually indicates a patient's dissatisfaction with treatment and an intention to sue for negligence.

The first reaction is one of anger, because you know that unless there is an obvious mistake on your part, you have tried your best to treat the patient satisfactorily. Then you start questioning your abilities and your confidence hits rock bottom. The telephone call to the Dental Defence Society, our indemnity provider, is always reassuring. They know how you are feeling and they have the uncanny ability to put it all in perspective for you. I am not talking about criminal investigations here, that is a completely different scenario, and I have no sympathy for professional people who try to take advantage of their position. I am referring to cases where something may have gone wrong and the relationship with the patient has deteriorated.

Often by apologising to the patient and offering to correct the situation, the complaint can be dealt with in house. Sometimes, however, there may be financial motivation to encourage the patient to press forward with a claim. I tend to divide these issues into three sections: dentist's error, no case to answer, or a dispute which if not settled may end up in court. In all these eventualities, solicitors on both sides may be involved. The dentists have a torrid time, wracked with guilt and confidence at low ebb, while the patients may become embroiled with distressing court cases. The majority of cases are settled out of court, but sometimes expert witnesses may be called in by each side, and appear in court, where a judgement is given. There is a trend now for patients to go directly to the General Dental Council, (GDC) as this can avoid the use of solicitors. Receiving a letter from the GDC can also be an unpleasant experience in that they have greater disciplinary powers.

Every dentist has failures where, in spite of your best efforts, things go wrong. I have never taken out the wrong tooth, but I have had bad days when treatment does not go to plan.

Mr C came to see me for a simple root treatment on an upper front tooth. I had known the patient for some time and we had a good rapport. Root treatment involves cleaning out the nerve canal and after cleaning, inserting an inert material, gutta percha, and sealing it in position. Whilst cleaning out the inside root, the fine instrument that I was using (reamer) fractured, and despite my best efforts it stubbornly refused to move. This is not negligence; it is a complication of treatment, a risk which is explained to the patient before treatment. I referred the patient to a specialist in root canals, and he completed the treatment for me. Mr C stayed with me as a patient and fully understood and appreciated my efforts. There is no blame here but I remember having a sleepless night or two wondering if it was my fault with all the guilt that goes with it.

My first solicitor's letter came in the late 1970s from a patient who had had immediate dentures, that is extractions with the denture being fitted at the same time. All went well, except after three weeks the patient complained that the denture plate was now very loose. Now after extractions there is often considerable shrinkage and a new lining on the denture or a replacement is needed. The patient, when informed of this, became quite aggressive and walked out, threatening to take legal action, which is exactly what he did. Sure enough, days later came the solicitor's letter claiming negligence, based on the fact that he claimed that he was not pre-warned that a replacement plate could be needed. No matter how much you know that this was not true, the deep feeling of anxiety always rears its ugly head. I contacted my protection society and sent them the patient's records.

In his records it clearly stated that he was warned that a reline or replacement was probably going to be required and also that he was given written instructions after the extractions. Case dropped by his solicitor, which should have been the end of it, but no, a few weeks later he was seen hurling a stone through the surgery window. Police involved. Not an awe-inspiring experience for me, the staff and the broken window. (Disaster.)

In the early 1980s I had completed a lower bridge for a regular patient who had never had any problem. For some reason the bridge completely failed after two years and fractured into two pieces, which meant that a new bridge was to be made at no cost to the patient. Appointments were made by him but he never arrived for them. This always arouses suspicion, especially when he failed to return telephone calls. Two weeks later the solicitor's letter arrived claiming negligence, pain and suffering, of course. Again, all my scrupulous records were sent to my insurers and I received a very reassuring letter that I had done all I could and that I had undoubtedly apologised to the patient for the technical failure of the bridge. The fact that I offered to replace it pro bono was noted. The case was settled without any admission of negligence, it being just an unfortunate occurrence, but, as is often the case in these situations, I assume he was remunerated for his suffering and distress.

I had booked in a local solicitor for some replacement crowns and we had allocated most of the morning to complete the job. This would involve removing all the old crowns, taking impressions and putting temporary covers on them. However, on the day, he failed to arrive in spite of a reminder. My manageress phoned him and politely asked why he had failed and didn't let us know. The reply was a curt, "I was too busy." Two weeks later he phoned for an appointment as one of the old crowns had fractured. Divine retribution, I thought. He came in and immediately turned to my manageress and accused her of being rude on the telephone. At that point I had to intervene and told him that I was present at the conversation and she was not rude. I then moved towards him saying that what was rude was him failing to attend a two- hour appointment, saying he was too busy to attend. I think he took my move towards him as an aggressive action and fled downstairs and out of the building. We never saw him again, but this demonstrates that sometimes, in what low esteem we as dentists are held.

You would not have thought that the war in Yugoslavia, 1998-1999, would in any way impinge on my NHS surgery in north Manchester. However, many of the refugees from Kosovo became temporary residents in my area and I was asked if I would provide dental treatment for them. We agreed, of course, but what followed was totally unexpected. Many came into the surgery with their families, but we only had one interpreter, which made communication very difficult. Although we reserved special days for treatment, the sheer number of patients was overwhelming. Their dental health was very poor, but worse was their overall medical condition. They were completely traumatised, some with obvious psychological problems, their eyes glazed and many with malnutrition. This was the first time I had seen people from a war zone, an experience that I could never forget. We did all we could dentally, but their problems were multifaceted, with some being referred straight to hospital. All the refugees thanked us but I felt that we had achieved very little, and then they were gone. (Disaster.)

It's always nice to be thanked by a patient and sometimes they are very generous, bringing in chocolates or biscuits, and it becomes difficult to refuse without causing offence. Mrs B ran an animal sanctuary and had neglected her teeth for many years. After the initial examination, it was agreed that she needed several roots extracting and some porcelain veneers. These are very thin pieces of shaped porcelain that can be used to change the shape or colour of teeth without removing too much enamel. The extractions proved to be very difficult and required surgical removal, that is lifting a flap of the gum around the teeth and removing some bone support, so that the roots could then be elevated. Eventually we completed the treatment and put in some stitches. Healing was uneventful and we then completed the porcelain veneers, which looked excellent. We all thought the improvement was significant. Mrs B was delighted with the result, but kept saying that the extractions had caused her considerable pain, so if she had known, she might not have had them done. Although it is normal to explain the possible complications associated with any treatment, in this case it was omitted in the patient's records. Obviously, we apologised and emphasised that perhaps, in the future, if she looked after her teeth better, she would avoid this happening again. There was no response to this but she did seem quite subdued when she left the surgery.

About a week later an aerated box arrived from her, together with a note saying, surprisingly, that she was now fine and in appreciation she wanted to give me a special Russian rabbit for my children. Okay, I thought a rabbit is easy to look after, so I peeped into the box and found an aggressive black rabbit trying desperately to escape.

The kids at home were delighted so we purchased a rabbit hutch and welcomed our new family member. The next day the 'beast from the east' escaped by kicking through the wooden hutch. I retrieved it and was scratched badly before I managed to put it back in and repair the hutch. The children would not go anywhere near it. Rasputin, as we called it, snarled and kicked its way around the garden, not the gentile fluffy rabbit I had anticipated. The final straw came when our neighbours' Alsatian came into our garden to look at the new visitor. Rasputin ran straight at the poor dog, which leapt back over the fence whimpering. "That's it," I informed the family and took it to the park, where we assume it became the local godfather.

We never saw Mrs B again, but I think schadenfreude? (Disaster.)

The General Dental Council (GDC)

The function of the GDC is defined by and governed by the Dentists Act 1984, which set out the following objectives.

1. To protect, promote and maintain the health, safety and well-being of the public.
2. To promote and maintain confidence in the dental profession.
3. To promote and maintain proper professional standards and conduct for members of those professions.

Unfortunately, there has been a trend for some members of the public to complain directly to the GDC, avoiding the need for solicitors' fees and inflicting more stress on the often-innocent dentist. Indeed, one spring morning in 2005 I was sitting at my desk at home opening my mail, and amongst all the other items that I had to deal with was a large brown envelope from the GDC. Heart rate up, anxiety level raised, and with trepidation I opened it.

'Your fitness to practise has been questioned.' These were the only words I can remember reading because it was nearly a mortal blow to my confidence and self-esteem. After a few moments these feelings were replaced by anger, both at the GDC and the patient. The GDC had given no thought to the well-being of the dentist, but in my opinion, seemed to imply that you were guilty until proven innocent, even though the patient's accusations were completely groundless.

I had started a lower bridge for Ms. D about six months earlier, and the preparations went smoothly. Impressions were taken and temporary crowns fitted. At this time, I had a camera so it was easy to take photographs to help with the records. Unfortunately, the patient had to go to America on business and cancelled the appointment for the final fitting. I heard nothing from her for the next two months, then a letter arrived saying that when she was in the gym where she was living, she had slipped, fallen and damaged her bridge. The letter was very apologetic, and promised to contact us as soon as possible. Efforts to call the patient were unsuccessful.

Then came the bombshell from the GDC. Granted they did not know the facts, but they produced a letter from the patient saying that the bridge that I had fitted failed and she was questioning my abilities. Yes, the GDC have a responsibility to patients, but also to the profession they represent. I took all the notes to my indemnity society, and their reaction was one of disbelief. They dealt with it from thereon and explained to all parties that the bridge that she had damaged was in fact temporary and that she had not returned to have the permanent bridge fitted. I felt that my abilities had been questioned, and was caused considerable despair by the false accusation. Added to this her fees were outstanding and it is clear to see why I was so angry and frustrated.

To their credit, the GDC asked the patient to come in for an examination but interestingly they never heard from her again. Eventually the case was dropped, with no case to answer. I was, incidentally, left with a very costly bridge made and ready to fit. This was not a pleasant experience which affected me badly for some months. It was the second time in my career that I had been seriously damaged emotionally, this time by a completely spurious allegation. However, it is important to concede that the GDC has a difficult job dealing with serious breaches of acceptable behaviour, sometimes criminal, so for an innocent dentist to be confronted with this scenario should be viewed with great caution and sensitivity.

Chapter Twenty-Five
Did They Just Build Pyramids?

Now for a brief lesson in ancient history…

St Apollonia

It was during the Roman period that toothache sufferers gained their own patron saint. Apollonia was the daughter of a magistrate in Alexandria who stood up for her Christianity, determined to save fellow Christians from persecution.

Dionysius, an Athenian judge and a Christian convert, says 'a mob… broke her teeth and threatened to burn her alive'. As she was being consumed by the fire, she called out that those who suffered from toothache and invoked her name would be relieved of their suffering. Around the year 300 she was made a saint by the Catholic Church and, because of her traumatic association with broken and damaged teeth, she is now known as the patron saint of dentistry. Who knew?

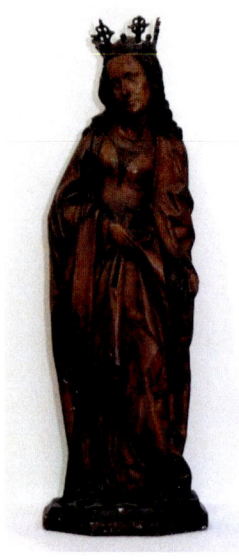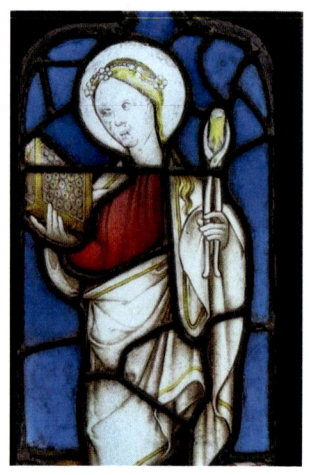

APOLLONIA PATRON SAINT OF DENTISTS
(*Photographs reproduced with the kind permission of
the British Dental Association museum*).

Prayer for Toothache to Saint Apollonia
(For use as a last resort)

O Glorious Apollonia, patron saint of dentistry and refuge to all those suffering from diseases of the teeth, I consecrate myself to thee, beseeching thee to number me among thy clients.

Dentistry in Ancient Egypt

I was not there, but there are some very interesting facts I would like to expand on.

Ancient recipes for toothpaste survive with ingredients such as bones, egg shells, pumice and myrrh, although there is no mention of toothbrushes.

The Greeks used mint, still a familiar ingredient in toothpaste for us today.

Early cures for toothache may seem strange to us. The Ancient Egyptians wore amulets, whilst the Roman writer, Pliny, recommended finding a frog by moonlight and asking it to take away your toothache.

A further cure, according to Scribonius Largus, doctor to the Emperor Claudius in the first century, involved 'fumigations made with the seeds of the Hyoscyamus [a poisonous plant known as 'stinking nightshade'] scattered on burning charcoal... followed by rinsings of the mouth with hot water, in this way... small worms are expelled'. The belief that cavities are caused by toothworms, is a longstanding one, held by the Ancient Egyptians and right up to the seventeenth century. If these cures seem bizarre, we should remember some modern similarities: a mouthrinse for the tongue in Ancient Egypt contained honey, just the same as our cure for a sore throat. (*Reproduced with kind permission of British Dental Association Museum, Ancient dentistry*).

The earliest recorded dentist not just in Egypt but in the world was Hesyre (Fig 1), who is evidenced from six exquisitely carved wooden panels that were found in his tomb at Saqqara near modern day Cairo, and which are generally considered to be the finest wood artefacts handed down from antiquity. Hesyre, who lived in about 2660 BC, was not only chief of dentists but also chief of physicians, as well as holding a number of other religious and secular titles. Other dentists similarly held multiple titles such as Nyanksekhmet, who was also a 'chief of physicians' and Khuwy who was not only a dentist, but 'elder of the physicians of the palace' as well as specialising in gastrointestinal complaints. Whether these multiple titles indicated that the individual was engaged in several specialities or that the titles were perhaps administrative or ceremonial is unclear, but overall, they do suggest a need for dental care.

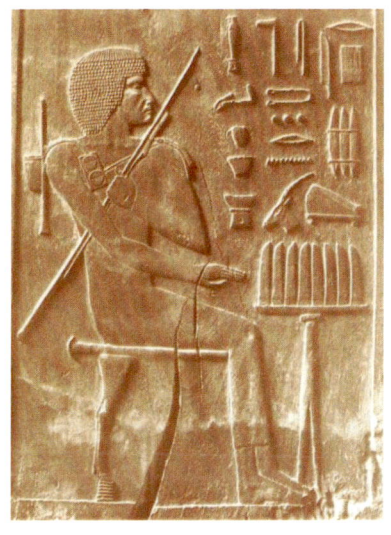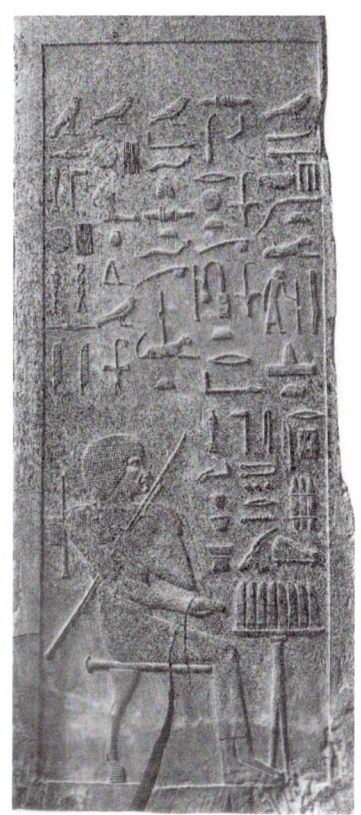

Fig 1 HESYRE, THE EARLIEST RECORDED
DENTIST

Look at how dentists from the time of the pharaohs applied practical knowledge in the field of dental, medicine and oral surgery

Of the so-called 'prosthetic appliances' that have been documented from ancient Egypt, the best-known example consists of a mandibular second molar connected by gold wire to a worn third molar (Fig. 2). It was discovered at Giza, near Cairo, in a burial shaft dating to approximately 2,500 BC and importantly, not found attached to a skull. The dental report at the time, which has since been questioned, stated that judging by the colour and anatomic form of the teeth they belonged to the same individual. Additionally, as the roots of the third molar were very absorbed, due to a probable inflammatory process, the tooth had become mobile, and so in an attempt to stabilise it, it had been attached to its neighbouring tooth.

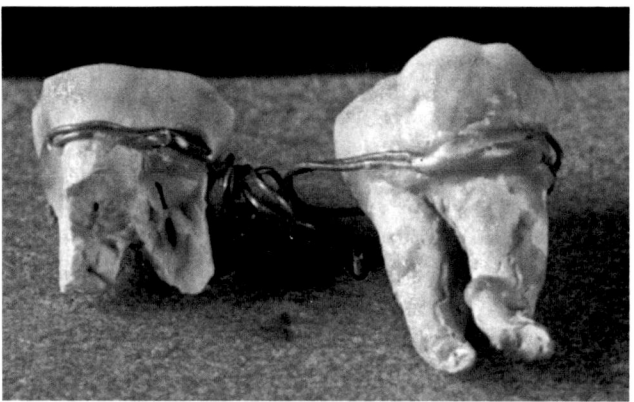

Fig.2 THE GIZA BRIDGE

A second appliance, similarly dated to about 2,500 BC, was excavated at el-Quatta, near Cairo and again was not found *in situ*, but retrieved from amongst the crushed bones of a skull (Fig. 3).

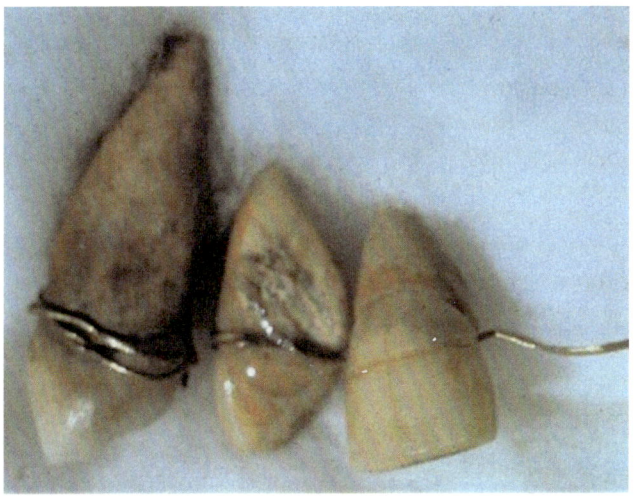

Fig 3 'EL-QUATTA BRIDGE'

Due to the flimsy nature of both these 'devices' they would not have been able to function during life. The gold tubular wire on the 'Giza device' was only 0.35mm thick. One possibility is that the devices were inserted into the mummied bodies in order to make them whole to enter the afterlife, a commonly held belief in ancient Egypt. False eyes and limbs have similarly been found on mummified remains.

Heavy tooth wear was typical for almost all the inhabitants of the land of the pharaohs. The primary cause of this tooth wear was the chewing throughout life of a coarse fibrous diet, made even more abrasive by the introduction of sand, particularly into the bread, the staple food of the ancient Egyptians. Excavated skulls and jaws show that the teeth condition is very bad—they are highly worn. By itself it is not a disease, but it is the basis for the rapid emergence of other more serious problems such as abscesses, inflammation of the gums and jaw bone and tooth loss.

The Edwin Smith papyrus is a well written and sophisticated example of medical literature, being the earliest known treatise dealing with surgery. This papyrus lists forty-eight mainly trauma cases and amongst them is one in which instructions are given for correcting a dislocated mandible: 'If you examine a man having a dislocation in his mandible [and] you find his mouth open [and] cannot close it for him, you should place your thumbs upon the ends of the two rami [lower jaw angles] in the inside of this mouth [and] your two groups of fingers under his chin, and you should cause them to fall back so that they rest in their place.'

It shows a clear logical approach differing little from the method that is practised today and importantly is the earliest description of a surgical procedure still in use.

There are probably no instruments so far excavated which can definitely be considered to have been used for dental purposes, but one difficulty in identification of any such instruments is that they were never engraved with their purpose. An example that has been suggested which may show dental instruments is a large scene inscribed on one of the walls of the temple of Kom-Ombo (Fig 4).

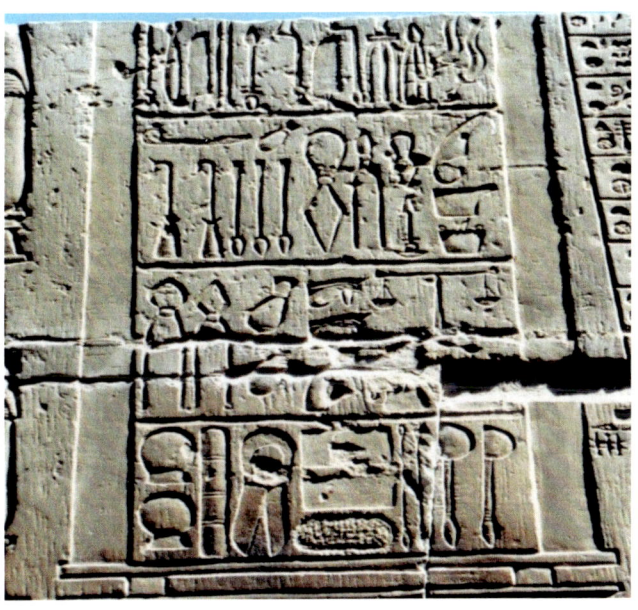

Fig 4 ANCIENT SURGICAL INSTRUMENTS?

Three prescriptions deal with oral pain and among the various components used to treat the condition was willow. Willow bark contains salicin, a chemical similar to acetylsalicylic acid, (aspirin), therefore having both analgesic and anti-inflammatory effects, although there is some doubt if the ancient Egyptians had discovered the true value of this plant.

Also of note, is that the Edwin Smith papyrus contains the first recorded use of absorbent lint made from vegetable fibre whilst splints and bandages are routinely used. It describes the use of adhesive strips in dealing with wounds, and cases of complex suturing are described in detail. It is clear from this papyrus that surgery was known, understood and practised in Ancient Egypt and that some of this knowledge is still in use today.

There is no evidence that the Ancient Egyptians filled teeth and no teeth have survived with any trace of materials being used as a filling.

Perhaps no discussion of medical and dental practice in Ancient Egypt could be complete without considering the part that magic played in the various prescriptions in the papyri. Certainly, the Ancient Egyptians were intelligent observers and discovered empirically some effective drugs and rational healing methods, but magic undoubtedly had a part to play. (*BDJ Published: 09 May 2009 R. J. Forshaw The practice of dentistry in ancient Egypt*).

Whilst we must give credit to the Ancient Egyptian dentists, and wonder at the materials they found to use, I can't help thinking that the prayers and spells were probably more affordable for the average person of the time. Even now, I sometimes give a silent prayer that the day goes without a hitch, and I can certainly think of the odd patient that I'd like to cast a spell on.

Chapter Twenty-Six
Emergencies

We are trained to deal with emergencies in the dental surgery. We practise CPR (cardiopulmonary resuscitation), and other scenarios. The most common emergency is syncope, a faint. This can usually be dealt with by putting the chair flat and administering oxygen if necessary. Over many years I knew that this particular emergency was caused by patients' extreme anxiety, and can often be avoided. To overcome their fear, I would spend a portion of the appointment time just sitting, talking and putting the patient at ease. I even had one man who insisted on telling me every detail of his current girlfriend and their problems before we commenced treatment. Occasionally a more serious emergency arose and this is where training and staff support count.

A patient came in for a routine filling appointment, with no medical problems. About half way through the procedure, she began to shake and we realised she was having an epileptic fit. The nurse collected the appropriate emergency box and we allowed the patient to recover on her own. We did not need to administer any medication and we did advise the patient to go and see her GP. Two weeks later we received a letter to say she had been diagnosed with a brain tumour, but it was anticipated that after surgery she would make a full recovery.

Although most emergencies can be avoided by reviewing the medical history of the patient, and planning for any possible problem, in this case there was no indication that the patient had any major underlying medical issues. Mrs J came to see me for a routine extraction. She had some heart trouble but she told us that she was not taking any medication. The extraction was uneventful but the bleeding would not stop. After five minutes I asked the patient again if she was taking any tablets. "I'm sorry. I'm taking warfarin but didn't want to tell you in case it stopped you taking the tooth out." Warfarin is an anti-coagulant, a blood thinner, and careful checks with the GP are required if a patient on this drug needs an extraction. After three stitches I managed to stop the bleeding and explained to the patient the risks she had taken.

It cannot always be assumed that a patient has given a complete medical history. There may be just a simple omission, but the dangers are there and in any invasive surgical procedure, vigilance is vital.

There is nothing funny about emergencies in the surgery; they can be frightening and unexpected. More often than not, the patient is very embarrassed and apologetic after any such event, and must be handled with sympathy and understanding.

Thank goodness I have never been in a situation where I have had to consider CPR for a patient, or indeed in any other scenario. However, one of my friends had to attend to a suspected heart attack outside a football stadium. I spoke to him afterwards and he was in a state of shock. He did everything correctly but still the man died. At that time there was no defibrillator close by which, if used, can dramatically improve the chances of survival. It is now standard practice today to have a defibrillator in the surgery and to be trained in its use.

Chapter Twenty-Seven
Goodbye, NHS

I had been working in the NHS for over forty years. During this period, I had seen all that is good and bad in the system. In the early days we had freedom in where we were to practise, and the type of dentistry we wanted to do, although we were restricted in some more complex cases which needed prior approval for certain treatments, such as multiple crowns and bridges. The system has evolved to become more basic and has become more expensive for patients. When I first started there was a flat rate fee of one pound fifty to pay. Now with the UDA system (Units of Dental Activity) there are to date three bands, with patient fees ranging from £22.70 to £269.30. So clearly, it is no longer a cheap system, although many people are exempt from fees. Because each dentist is now restricted to a certain number of UDAs, after they are completed there is no incentive or payment to continue with treatments. In this way, in my opinion, the NHS keeps a tight rein on the cost of the dental services.

Is it underfunded? Yes, of course, like many other areas of the NHS. Remember, however, dental decay and its associated problems is the most prevalent disease. Unmet dental needs and untreated dental decay represent a significant disease burden for children and adults.

The two main types of dental disease are: tooth decay (dental caries or cavities) and gum disease (periodontal disease). Both can cause pain, infection and loss of teeth if left untreated.

Dental decay

This is probably the most common health problem in the UK, although the incidence has been reducing, but still almost half of the population do not attend a dentist. Shockingly, tooth decay remains the leading reason for hospital admissions among five to nine-year-olds, according to data published by NHS Digital. The number of admissions for tooth decay was more than double those for acute tonsillitis, which is the second highest cause of hospital admissions for this age group. Figures for children aged five to nine in 2018-2019 show 25,702 hospital admissions for tooth decay, and 11,811 admissions for acute tonsillitis. For age one to four there were nearly 7,000 admissions, and these children may be having extractions under general anaesthetic which always has risk and can be traumatic. Many days of school are missed because of these tooth related problems.

Tooth decay can be prevented by education, fluoride toothpaste and regular attendance at dentists, together with alteration in diet, particularly a decreased sugar consumption. It is estimated that children and young adults aged eleven to eighteen consume the equivalent of a bathtub full of sugary drinks every year; those aged four to ten, about half a bathtub. Dental treatment for the under eighteens is free of charge, although there can be difficulty accessing dental care in some parts of the country. *(With kind permission of the Royal College of Surgeons of England).*

Periodontal disease

This affects the gums, bone and other supporting tissues of the teeth. Although most individuals suffer gum inflammation from time to time, around ten percent of the population appear to suffer from the more severe forms of the disease, which cause loss of supporting bone. This group appears to be at greatest risk of losing teeth through periodontal disease. It is caused by the bacteria which regularly collect on the teeth.

Periodontal disease is a very common condition where the gums become swollen, sore or infected. Most adults in the UK have gum disease to some degree, and most people experience it at least once, though it is much less common in children. The early stage of gum disease is known as gingivitis (early inflammation of the gums). If not treated, a condition called periodontitis can develop. This affects the tissues that support teeth and hold them in place. If periodontitis is neglected, the bone in the jaw may be damaged and small spaces between the teeth can open, leading to tooth loss.

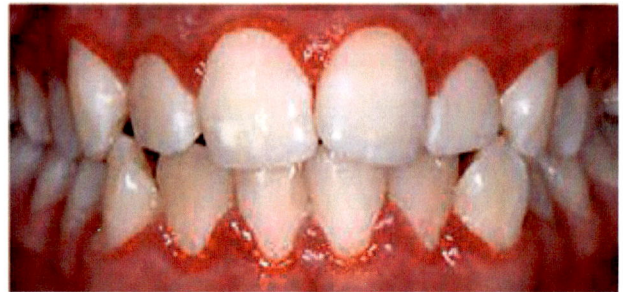

Gingivitis

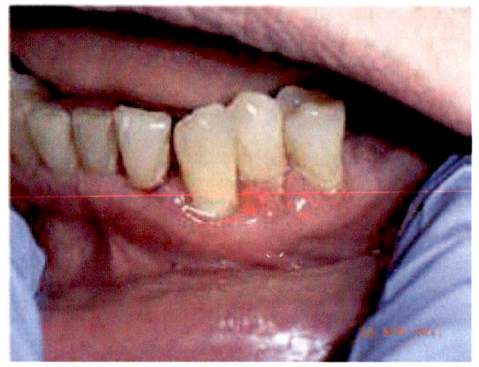

Peridontitis

(Kind permission of the British Society of Periodontology and Implant dentistry).

With this in mind, we as dentists have been fighting an uphill struggle to keep pace not only with the amount of dental disease, but also the cost to the country of dealing with the consequences. Then we had further regulations from the CQC (Care Quality Commission) overseeing how we operate. I can remember now spending several thousand pounds on a washer disinfector machine, only to find out later that we did not really need one. The work of the NHS is massive and the CQC must be given credit for trying to keep all our patients safe and treated in the correct environment.

After forty years of battling with these issues, it was time for me to leave the NHS, and in a very tearful and emotional afternoon I handed over my staff and surgery to their new owner who has gone from strength to strength and is still treating most of the original patients. I said farewell to NHS dentistry and continued to work in my private surgery, but was able to keep in touch with the wonderful patients and staff that had been such an important part of my life.

The NHS is, in my opinion, an excellent and unique system, where patients should be able to access oral health advice and dental treatment wherever they live. However, this is not always so because of the restrictions imposed on dentists at present. Contracts are in the gift of the local authority, and, due to financial limitations, are not always available.

Chapter Twenty-Eight
The Corporate Challenge

At the private rooms, there was only a handful of the original directors and tenants still in residence. We were all getting older and retirement was looming. Bev and I were still beavering away and the practice continued to be very busy. It was, however, getting more difficult for the single-handed practitioner to continue operating. There were more and more regulations and we spent a substantial amount of surgery time dealing with non-surgical matters.

One Friday morning in August 2015, I received a letter from one of the corporates that ran many surgeries, asking me if I wished to sell my practice and move to a multi-surgery not too far away. I knew the people there well and realised that this was a good escape strategy, leading ultimately to retirement. I discussed it with Bev, my manageress, who had been with me from the beginning, and we decided to accept. Every patient was informed and given directions to our new home. To leave my beautiful rooms, where I was beholden to nobody, was a terrible wrench, but I knew that this was the way forward.

In February 2016 we moved everything, contents and chair to the new place, and again we had to say goodbye to a building that had been our life for forty years. This was a very sad time, as the building held many wonderful memories and ghosts from the past. Those brilliant people who worked in the buildings, the consultants, the staff, and all the laughter and sad times we shared, seemed to linger in the air as we left, but those days were gone and were now part of history. It was time to leave.

After being my own boss for decades, I was now working as an associate in a completely different environment, with different people and systems. It took only a few months for us to be fully integrated and soon it seemed as if we belonged.

Being part of a large corporate organisation has many benefits. So much that I was accustomed to doing, was now completed for me. Wages were paid, materials purchased and all the day to day running problems in the surgery were dealt with. All I had to do was treat my patients, and virtually all followed me to my new place of work.

This was a fitting way to complete my career; I started with no surgery of my own and finished in the same way; the wheel had come the full circle, with a few bumps in the road. (Triumph.)

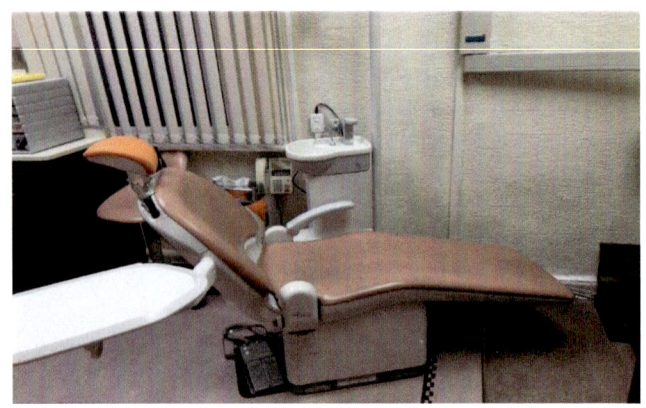

The chair ready to move

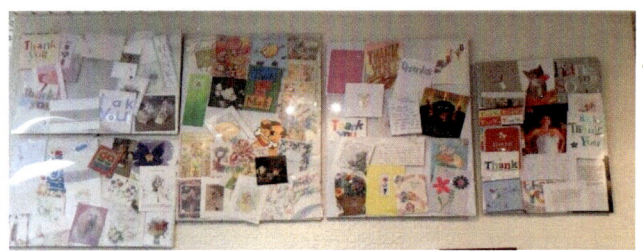

Oh, those thank you cards

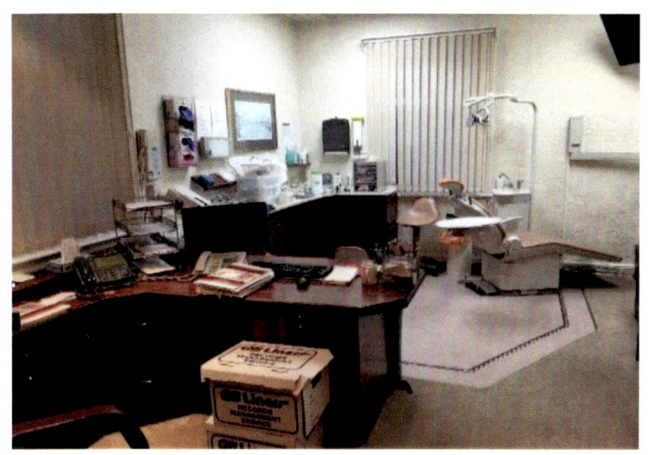

Packing up…

Chapter Twenty-Nine
Would I Do it all Again?

I am now sitting in my office staring blankly at my appointment book on the computer screen. I see lists of patients with familiar names, and I can picture the families, the grandparents, parents and children. I can hear them talking about their lives, their holidays, personal problems as well as their dental issues, and you know what? I feel flattered and honoured that I have been able to touch so many people's lives.

That I have had more triumphs than disasters is so important to me as I look at the thankyou cards and letters of appreciation from grateful patients. Rudyard Kipling, eat your heart out. Then I look at my appointment book again, and move it forward to my retirement day, and beyond that it's grey and blanked off as if the world will end on that day and there is no future.

Well, it doesn't, it's just another completed chapter in my life. Would I do it all again, meet and work with such a myriad of personalities, a microcosm of the world, and make a difference? Of course I would! (Triumph!)